CMOS IC Design for Wireless Medical and Health Care

Zhihua Wang • Hanjun Jiang • Hong Chen

CMOS IC Design
for Wireless Medical
and Health Care

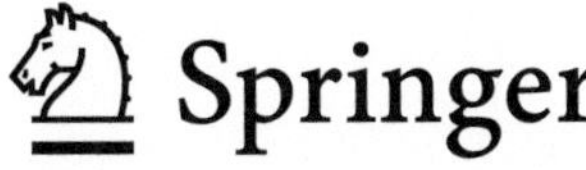 Springer

Zhihua Wang
Institute of Microelectronics
Tsinghua University
Beijing, People's Republic of China

Hanjun Jiang
Institute of Microelectronics
Tsinghua University
Beijing, People's Republic of China

Hong Chen
Institute of Microelectronics
Tsinghua University
Beijing, People's Republic of China

ISBN 978-1-4939-5486-5   ISBN 978-1-4614-9503-1 (eBook)
DOI 10.1007/978-1-4614-9503-1
Springer New York Heidelberg Dordrecht London

Preface

Since the invention of the first electronic general-purpose computer ENIAC in 1946, there have been great breakthroughs in the computing technologies, especially after the invention of semiconductor integrated circuit (IC) in 1958. The computer in 1946 occupied a big room and could be only operated by trained scientists and technicians. However, today's computers such as the tablets and smartphones can be put into the pocket with much higher computation capability, and can be easily used by every common people. What's behind the development of computers is a bunch of modern technologies, especially the semiconductor integrated circuits (ICs). For the past few decades, following the Moore's Law, advances in semiconductor ICs have been continuously pushing the development of computing technology towards miniaturization, intelligentialization, and informationization.

Many people have predicted that wellness-related industry and business will be the next focus of the global economy. The evolution of wellness depends on a few key factors, including the development of medical and health care technology. It is believed that the semiconductor ICs will bring the same story to the medical and health care technology, as what have happened to the computing technology. Actually, such changes have already taken place, with the aid of semiconductor ICs. For example, today's ECG acquisition device using ICs can stick to the chest like a bandage, while the first electrocardiography (ECG) equipment invented about 100 years ago weighed about 600 lb. However, due to the diversity of medical and health care applications, the continuous efforts from both the industry and academia are required to propel the development of the medical and health care technology, and to finally achieve the ubiquitous medical and health care.

About 15 years ago, our research group made a decision to choose the medical and health care electronics as one of the major research directions. Ever since then, we have conducted a number of research projects to apply the state-of-the-art CMOS IC techniques to the wireless medical and health care applications, such as the cochlear implants for hearing aid, capsules for gastrointestinal examinations, measurement devices for artificial joint replacement surgeries, neural stimulators, and human body sound monitoring. More than 300 technical papers have been published, and over 50 patents have been filed. Some research results transferred to industry have been commercialized or are being commercialized.

In these projects, we have investigated CMOS circuit design techniques, such as the biomedical sensor acquisition circuits, low power wireless transceivers, power management circuits, digital controllers, and system-on-a-chip (SoC) integration techniques, which are required to build the wireless medical/health care application systems. In this book, we will present the typical design techniques of these CMOS circuits, by taking the wireless capsule endoscope systems and the wireless ligament balance measuring system in total knee arthroplasty as the examples. The basic design considerations, the system level architectures, and the transistor level implementation will be discussed, to give the readers both the whole picture and the circuit details.

We have just experienced the great era of information technology which has reshaped the economy and society in an unprecedented manner. We believe that we will also witness the new era of ubiquitous medical and health care in the coming future, on the foundation of semiconductor integrated circuits and other modern technologies. The development of wireless and health care application systems using CMOS integrated circuits are making progress towards miniaturization, intelligentialization, and informationization. It is our honor to make some contribution to this great evolution by writing this book.

Beijing, People's Republic of China   Zhihua Wang
                                                                            Hanjun Jiang
                                                                            Hong Chen

Acknowledgements

The content of this book is based on the research work accomplished by the Integrated Circuits and System (ICAS) group of Tsinghua University, Beijing, China. The professors and graduate students in ICAS group have made significant technical contributions to the content of this book. The technical contributors are listed below.

- Ziqiang Wang, assistant professor of Tsinghua Univ.
- Xu Zhang, former postdoctoral researcher of ICAS, now with Institute of Semiconductor, Chinese Academy of Science.
- Fule Li, associate professor of Tsinghua Univ.
- Xiang Xie, associate professor at Tsinghua Univ.
- Baoyong Chi, associate professor of Tsinghua Univ.
- Chun Zhang, associate professor of Tsinghua Univ.
- Woogeun Rhee, professor of Tsinghua Univ.
- Dongmei Li, associate professor of Tsinghua Univ.
- Guolin Li, associate professor of Tsinghua Univ.
- Songping Mai, associate professor of Shenzhen Graduate School of Tsinghua Univ.
- Lingwei Zhang, former Ph. D. student of ICAS, now with GalaxyCore Inc.
- Xinkai Chen, former Ph. D. student of ICAS, now with Ecore Technologies, Ltd.
- Xiaoyu Zhang, former Ph. D. student of ICAS, now with VIA Technologies, Inc.
- Hui Jiang, former master student of ICAS, now Ph. D. student of TU Delft
- Yanqing Ning, former Ph. D. student of ICAS, now with Ecore Technologies, Ltd.
- Ming Liu, former Ph. D. student of ICAS, now with Institute of Semiconductor, Chinese Academy of Science.
- Shuguang Han, former Ph. D. student of ICAS, now with Institute of Semiconductor, Chinese Academy of Science.
- Liyuan Liu, former Ph. D. student of ICAS, now with Institute of Semiconductor, Chinese Academy of Science.

The authors would also show thanks to the scientists and engineers of Ecore Technologies Ltd., at Beijing and Hitron Technologies Ltd., at Hangzhou, for their great effort to commercialize the research results.

Contents

Chapter 1
Introduction

1.1 Emerging Wireless Medical and Health Care Applications

Nowadays, with the economic development and social evolution, people are paying more and more attention on the life quality with an increasing demand on wellness. As pointed out by Paul Zane Pilzer pointed out in his book *"the New Wellness Revolution: How to Make a Fortune in the Next Trillion Dollar Industry,"* the next big thing is the wellness revolution [1].

The demand on wellness is increasing with several facts:

1. The world's population is living longer. As shown in Fig. 1.1 [2], the mean age of death for people all the global areas has shown evident growth in the past 40 years. For example, the average death age in East Asia has increased to 66 years in 2010, compared to 36 years in 1970. Actually, since 1970, the average age of death has increased 35 years [2]. The increasing population of aged people has raised the huge challenge of the entire human society. In the other hand, this change has also brought a great opportunity for the development of technologies and economic. With this change, people have seen both the challenge and the opportunity for the wellness industry.
2. With the global economic development, the human society is now in the wealthiest period in the history. The world has accumulated enormous fortune in the past few decades. With such an economic base, people in the developed countries and emerging countries now can move their focus to the life quality so that the wellness revolution is a must.
3. There has been great technology progress in the past one century, including material science, information technologies, biology, mechanic engineering, etc. The technology development has made it possible to produce all kinds of powerful equipment to fulfill the human needs, including the need on wellness.

The emergence and development of new medical and health care equipment is one of the major forces driving the wellness revolution. In the past a few decades,

Z. Wang et al., *CMOS IC Design for Wireless Medical and Health Care,*
DOI 10.1007/978-1-4614-9503-1_1, © Springer Science+Business Media New York 2014

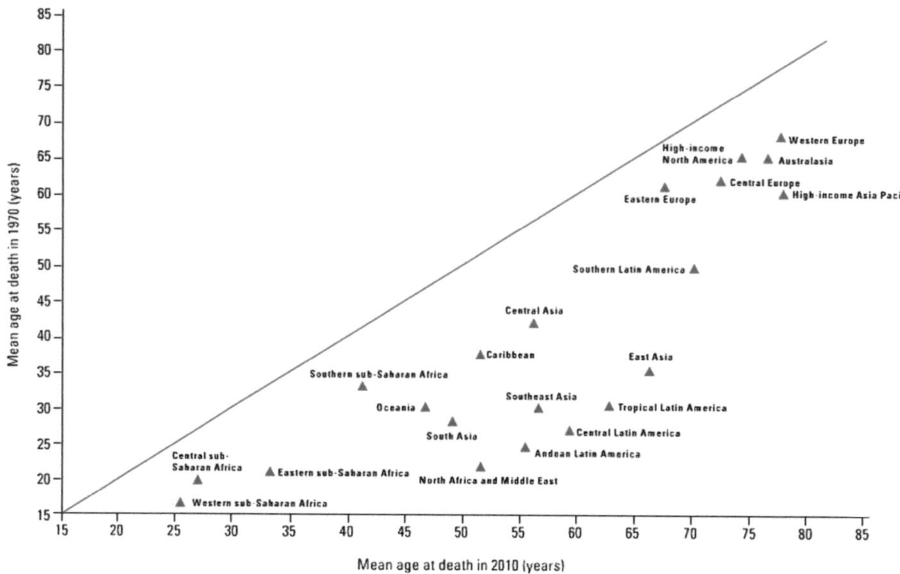

Fig. 1.1 Mean age of death, 1970 compared with 2010, Institute for Health Metrics and Evaluation, The Global Burden of Disease: Generating Evidence, Guiding Policy, Seattle, WA: IHME, 2013

with the development of microelectronics, integrated circuits, micromechanics, and material technologies, there have been great progress in medical electronics. Scientists and engineers from the industry and academia have been working together to create some new medical and health care equipment that only existed in the science fictions in the past, such as:

- Cochlear implants for hearing aid [3, 4]
- Capsule endoscope for gastrointestinal tract examination [5–8]
- Artificial arm and leg prosthesis [9–11]
- Implantable visual prosthesis [12, 13]
- Artificial heart pacemaker [14]
- Urinary incontinence prosthesis [15]
- Brain–computer interface [16]
- Wireless body sensors measuring pressure, pH, temperature sensors, etc. [17–19]

These new medical and health care systems are featured with high integration level, advanced intelligence, reliability and safety and can perform the functions of information acquisition, signal processing, wireless communication, etc. They can be used to help the doctors for disease diagnosis and treatment and to help the patent to rebuild some physical functions. These systems also drive the new wellness revolution by shifting the traditional sickness-oriented medical and health care to the new prevention-oriented medical and health care (Fig. 1.2).

Today, with the development of communication technologies, information technology, mobile internet, etc., the wireless communication turns to be one of the

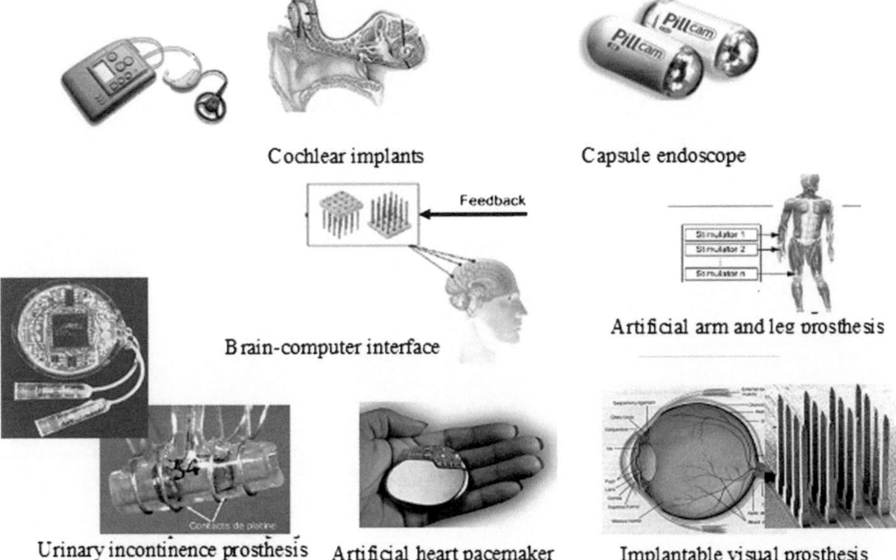

Fig. 1.2 Typical emerging medical and health care systems

major features of the emerging medical and health care systems. The latest medical and health care products can be wireless connected to the internet through the mobile terminals. Some medical and health care products use the built-in hardware inside the mobile terminals with wireless connections, such as the heart rate detection software in the smartphones.

In general, the wireless medical and health care application systems, with the boost of those cutting-edge techniques including communication, internet, software, materials, and manufacturing, have emerged as an important part of the new wellness revolution.

1.2   Technology Trends

Before discussing the technology trends of the wireless medical and health care applications, it will be interesting to briefly take a look at the development history of modern computers.

In the past few decades, computers have greatly reshaped almost all the aspects of the human society and the daily life of everybody. Nowadays, people are using computers, all kind of dimensions and forms, from the supercomputers such as the Tianhe-2 in Guangzhou, China and the Titan in Oak Ridge, USA, to the tablet computers and pocket computers (smartphones), in almost every area and every action, including scientific research, engineering development, business, office work,

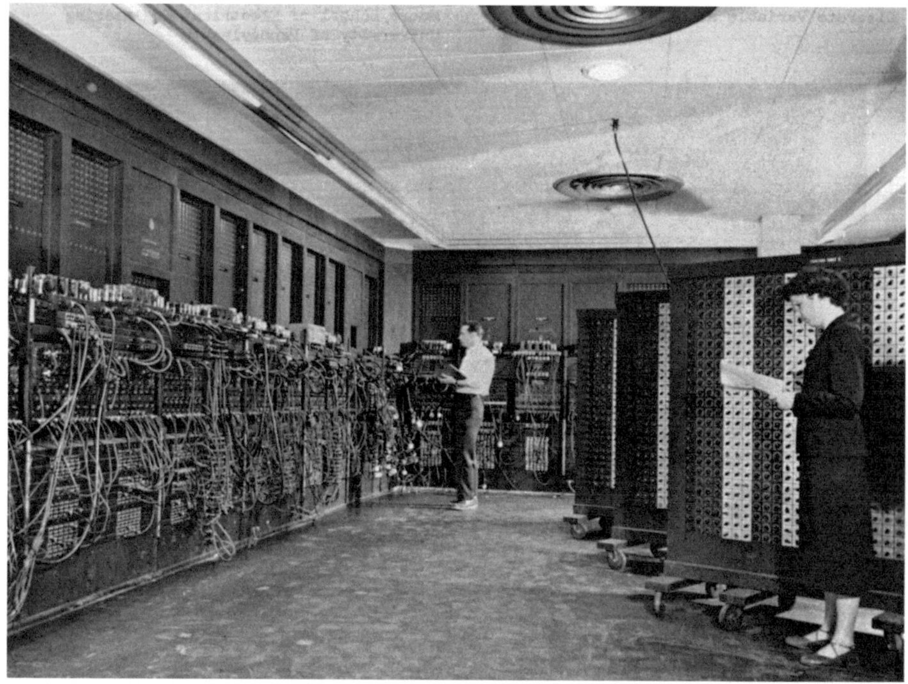

Fig. 1.3 ENIAC in Philadelphia, PA, available at http://www.wikipedia.com

knowledge learning, entertainment, etc. The computer technology is a representative of modern technologies and the base of many other technologies, and it will be found that the technology trends shown in the computer technology development is widely applicable to many other technologies, such as the medical and health care technology that will be the focus of this book.

It is well known that the first electronic general-purpose computer ENIAC (Electronic Numerical Integrator And Computer) was built in University of Pennsylvania in 1946, following many great pioneer creations such as the first non-programmable electronic digital computer ABC (Atanasoff-Berry Computer) by Iowa State University in 1939 and the first functional program-controlled Turing-complete computer Z3 created by Konrad Zuse in 1941. The ENIAC contained 17,468 vacuum tubes and quite many other components. It weighed about 30 tons, was roughly $2.4 \times 0.9 \times 30$ m, took up 167 m^2, and consumed 150 kW of power. It could perform 5,000 addition or subtraction operations per second [20]. Figure 1.3 shows the ENIAC, which occupied a large room.

There are a few remarkable milestones in the development history of computers in the next decades following ENIAC:

1. In 1953, the first transistorized computer was built at the University of Manchester [21]. This second-generation computer used transistors invented in 1947 to replace the vacuum tubes.

2. Starting from 1960s, the integrated circuits (ICs) invented by Jack Kilby in 1958 were used to build the third-generation computers with decreased size and cost while increased speed and reliability.
3. In 1971, Intel released the world's first commercial microprocessor Intel 4004 using the large-scale integration (LSI) microchip technology [22]. The microprocessor-based computers using LSI and later on the very-large-scale integration (VLSI) technology are recognized as the fourth-generation computers.
4. In 1973, the IBM Los Gatos Scientific Center developed a portable computer prototype called SCAMP (Special Computer APL Machine Portable), which was designated as "the world's first personal computer" by PC Magazine in 1983. The IBM 5100, the first commercially available portable computer, appeared in September 1975 and was based on the SCAMP prototype [23]. This began the great era of personal computer.
5. Nowadays, almost everybody has one or even multiple pocket computers, namely, the smartphones and tablet computers. The sale number of the smartphones and tablet computers exceeded that of personal computers in 2011 [24, 25]. The originally huge computer which occupied a big room can now be put in the pocket with much more powerful computation capability and much less power consumption.

In the road of computer development, we have seen three major trends:

1. Miniaturization: the first electronic general purpose ENIAC occupied several rooms, and then through the past 6 decades the computer was moved to the desktop, and the laptop, and finally the pockets.
2. Intelligentialization: the first computers could only be operated by the well-trained scientists and technicians, but nowadays even a teenage kid can easily use a tablet computer to search maps, shop online, and play games.
3. Informationization: with the internet and the mobile internet, almost all today's computers are connected, and people can easily share information at different levels, and the service providers can then offer various information services to every computer end user.

It has been observed that the development of computer has benefited from the development of semiconductor. What is behind the rapid development of computer after 1960s is the advancement of semiconductor integrated circuits. Since Intel co-found Gordon E. Moore proposed the Moore's Law [26] in 1965, which claimed that the number of components in integrated circuits would doubled every year, the complementary metal–oxide–semiconductor (CMOS) technology has followed the Moore's Law, though not that accurately, for almost 5 decades. In some sense, the semiconductor technology has been promoting the performance of computer towards miniaturization, intelligentialization, and informationization.

The same story is happening not just to computers, but to many other application areas. The electronic equipment for the medical and health care purpose has the same story. We can take a quick review on the development history of the electrocardiography (ECG) as the example.

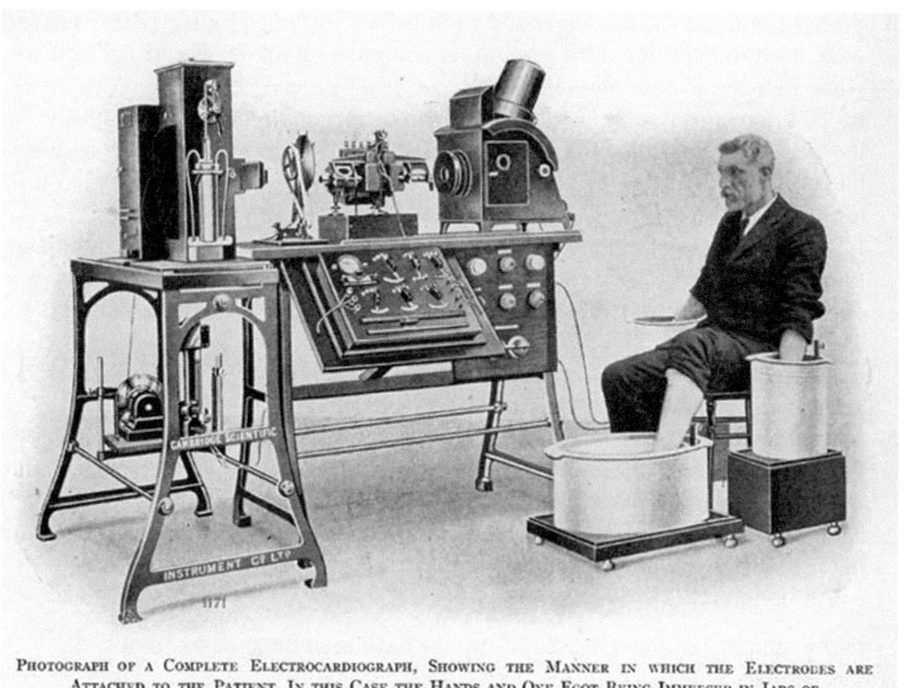

Fig. 1.4 The first table-model Einthoven ECG machine manufactured by the Cambridge Scientific Instrument Company of London in 1911 [29]

The attempt to capture the heart's electrical activity can be traced back to the eighteenth century. It is well known that the Dutch physiologist Willem Einthoven used the string galvanometer he invented in 1901 [27] to build the first modern ECG machine in 1902 [27]. Later on, Einthoven won a Nobel Prize in 1924 for his contributions to the field of ECG. The first Einthoven ECG machine weighted about 600 lb and required five people for operation [28]. Figure 1.4 shows the first table-model Einthoven ECG machine manufactured by the Cambridge Scientific Instrument Company of London in 1911 [29].

With the invention of the vacuum tube in 1900s, people began to use vacuum tubes to amplify the electrodiagram starting from 1920s [28]. This helped to reduce the ECG machine weight and move the ECG machine to a patient's bedside. The Cambridge Instrument Company built a device that weighed 50 lb; by 1935, the Sanborn Company had reduced the weight to 25 lb [27].

In 1949, the physicist Norman J. Holter invented the Holter monitor [30], which is a portable device for continuous ECG monitoring for a time period from 24 h to 2 weeks at a time. Built with integrated circuits, the dimension of today's Holter monitors, such as SuperECG company's HeartBug ECG monitor, can be down to $61 \times 46 \times 20$ mm^3 and weigh only 99 g [31].

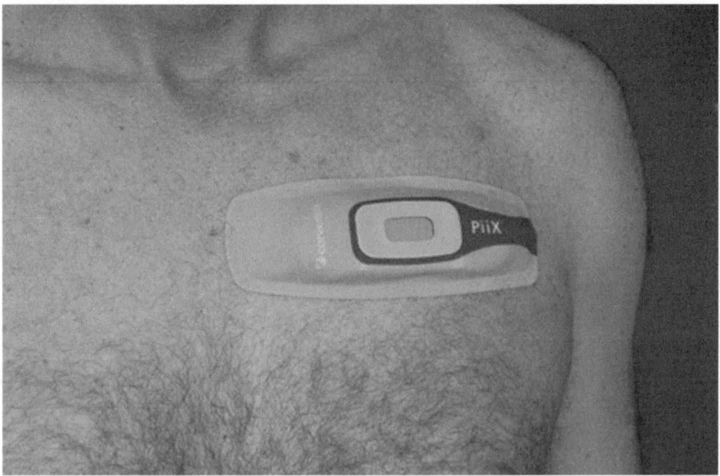

Fig. 1.5   Corventis company's wearable bandage-like ECG device [31]

The latest development of ECG equipment includes those wearable ECG devices. For example, Corventis company's NUVANT Mobile Cardiac Telemetry (MCT) System uses a wearable bandage-like device [32] as shown in Fig. 1.5, to capture ECG signals. AliveCor's ECG monitoring case for iPhone gets FDA approval in December, 2012. By attaching a case with two electrodes to the iPhone, the users can easily get the ECG waveforms by putting two fingers on the electrodes [33].

From the development history of ECG devices, the same trends can be observed for medical and health care products, as happened to computers.

1. Miniaturization: the medical and health care equipment was very hulking in the history. With the aid of electronics and microelectronics, nowadays people can produce very small medical and health care devices for the wearable or even implantable applications.
2. Intelligentialization: the old medical and health care equipment could only be operated by the well-trained doctors and technicians. By using single automatic control and processing techniques as well as the user-friendly software, the individuals can easily operate many medical and health care with following some simple instruction from the manufacturers and doctors.
3. Informationization: the emerging wireless medical and health care products can be connected to the internet wire/wirelessly via various networking connections. The information acquired can be stored, analyzed, and shared based on the cloud computing.

Again, there are many advanced technologies behind the development of wireless medical and health care applications. Among these technologies, the CMOS technology is one of the enabling technologies.

1.3   What to Expect in This Book

As can been in the previous section, the semiconductor integrated circuit (IC) technologies have been continuously boosting the development of computers, the medical/health care equipment, and many other technologies.

The silicon-based CMOS technology is one of the most important IC technologies. It is widely used to build analog amplifiers, data converters, microprocessors, microcontrollers, memories, and other circuits. ICs built using the CMOS technology have the features of low static power consumption and high noise immunity. Also, the CMOS technology has the important characteristic of scaling down [34], which makes the CMOS technology follow the Moore's Law in the past 5 decades with steady speed and complexity increasing, and cost and power consumption reduction. And the continuous improvement in CMOS technology has been one of the driving reasons for the rapid development of today's electronics systems and devices.

To implement a wireless medical/health care systems with the features of miniaturization, intelligentialization, and informationization using the CMOS technology, there are quite many challenges. The two most challenges are the integration level and the power consumption.

1. Integration level: to have a small form factor, especially for those implantable devices, the CMOS IC for wireless medical/health care applications should try to integrate all the functions within ICs as few as possible, and the best solution is to build a system-on-a-chip (SoC). Such a chipset or an SoC needs to have the functions of biomedical signal acquisition, microcontroller, digital signal processing, wireless transceiver, power management, etc. Also, to make the final device small, the designers should design a chipset/SoC using as few external components as possible.
2. Power consumption: wireless medical/health care devices, especially those implantable devices, are usually powered by tiny coin batteries. The chipset/SoC for these applications needs to have very low power consumption. Also, note that the batteries can be the limited factor for the device dimension; low power consumption means that the device can use small batteries with a certain battery life requirement so that the device size can be small.

This book will focus on the CMOS IC design techniques for wireless medical and health care applications, featured with high integration level and low power consumption. This book will give insight view of the design principles of CMOS IC for wireless medical and health care, based on two successfully commercialized design examples. Design techniques on both the circuit block level and the system level will be discussed, based on the real design examples investigated by the authors' research group. CMOS IC design techniques for the entire signal chain of wireless medical and health care systems will be covered, including biomedical signal acquisition, wireless transceiver, power management, and SoC integration, with the emphasis on the ultra-low-power IC design techniques.

The two design examples include the wireless capsule endoscope systems and the wireless ligament balance measuring system in total knee arthroplasty (TKA).

The following chapters of this book will be organized as follows:

The typical system architecture and the design considerations will be discussed in Chap. 2.

The CMOS IC design techniques for biomedical signal acquisition circuit, including the sensor interface circuit and the digitization circuit, will be presented in Chap. 3.

The low-power CMOS wireless transceiver design techniques for medical/health care applications will be discussed in Chap. 4, based on a few transceiver design examples.

Other important circuit design techniques, including the power management circuits and the low-power digital controller, will be presented in Chap. 5.

The SoC design techniques and application systems implementation details will be given in Chap. 6.

References

1. Pilzer PZ. The new wellness revolution: how to make a fortune in the next trillion dollar industry. 2nd ed. Hoboken, NJ: Wiley; 2007.
2. Institute for Health Metrics and Evaluation. The global burden of disease: generating evidence, guiding policy. Seattle, WA: IHME; 2013.
3. Germanovix W, Toumazou C. Design of a micropower current-mode log-domain analog cochlear implant. In: IEEE transactions on circuits and systems II: analog and digital signal processing, 2000. vol. 47. p. 1023–46.
4. Laizou PC. Signal-processing techniques for cochlear implants. IEEE Eng Med Biol Mag. 1999;18:34–46.
5. Iddan G, Meron G, Glukhovsky A, et al. Wireless capsule endoscopy. Nature. 2000;405: 417–8.
6. Palan B, Roubik K, Husak M, et al. CMOS ISFET-based structures for biomedical applications. In: 1st annual international conference on microtechnologies in medicine and biology, Lyon, France, 2000. p. 368–71.
7. Errachid A, Godignon P, Ivorra A, et al. Implementation of multisensor silicon needles for cardiac applications. In: CAS 2001 proceedings of the international semiconductor conference, USA, 2001. p. 222–5.
8. Park HJ, Nam HW, Song BS, et.al. Design of bi-directional and multi-channel miniaturized telemetry module for wireless endoscopy. In: 2nd annual international IEEE-EMB special topic conference on microtechnologies in medicine & biology, Madison, WI, 2002. p. 273–6.
9. Wessberg J, Stambaugh CR, et al. Real-time prediction of hand trajectory by ensembles of cortical neurons in primates. Nature. 2000;408:361–5.
10. Manal K, Gonzalez RV, Lloyd DG, et al. A real-time EMG-driven virtual arm. Comput Biol Med. 2002;32:25–36.
11. Nicolelis MAL. Actions from thoughts. Nature. 2001;409:403–7.
12. Schwarz M, Ewe L, Hijazi N, et al. Micro implantable visual prostheses. In: 1st annual international conference on microtechnologies in medicine and biology, Lyon, France, 2000. p. 400–3.
13. Zrenner E. Will retinal implants restore vision. Science. 2002;295:1022–5.

14. Wessels D. Implantable pacemakers and defibrillators: device overview & EMI considerations. In: IEEE international symposium on electromagnetic compatibility, USA, 2002. vol. 2. p. 911–5.
15. Mouine J, Brunner D, Chtourou Z. Design and implementation of a multichannel urinary incontinence prosthesis. In: Proceedings of the 22nd annual international conference of the IEEE Engineering in Medicine and Biology Society, Chicago, 2000. p. 321–4.
16. Jonathan RW, Niels B, William JH. Brain-computer interface technology: a review of the first international meeting. IEEE Trans Rehabil Eng. 2000;8:222–5.
17. Chatzandroulis S, Tsoukalas D, Neukomm PA. A miniature pressure system with a capacitive sensor and a passive telemetry link for use in implantable applications. J Microelectromech Syst. 2000;9:18–23.
18. Mackay RS, Jacobson B. Endoradiosonde. Nature. 1957;179:1239–40.
19. Zworkin VK. Radio pill. Nature. 1957;179:898.
20. Weik MH. A survey of domestic electronic digital computing systems. Ballistic Research Laboratories Report No. 971. US Department of Commerce, Dec 1955.
21. Lavington S. Early British computers. Manchester: Manchester University Press; 1980.
22. Intel 4004 microprocessor family. http://www.cpu-world.com
23. Before the beginning: Ancestors of the IBM personal computer. http://www-03.ibm.com/ibm/history/exhibits/pc/pc_1.html
24. Maier D. Sales of smartphones and tablets to exceed PBS. 2011. http://www.practicalecommerce.com/
25. Anderson DP, Kilburn T. A pioneer of computer design. IEEE Ann Hist Comput. 2009;31(2):84.
26. Moore GE. Cramming more components onto integrated circuits. Electronics. 1965;38(8):114–7.
27. Rivera-Ruiz M, Cajavilca C, Varon J. Einthoven's string galvanometer, the first electrocardiograph. Tex Heart Inst J. 2008;35(2):174–8.
28. Zywietz C. A brief history of electrocardiography—progress through technology. Hannover: Biosignal Institute for Biosignal Processing and Systems Research; 2003.
29. Burch GE, DePasquale NP. A history of electrocardiography. Chicago: Year Book Medical Publishers; 1964.
30. Hilbel T, Helms TM, Mikus G, Katus HA, Zugck C. Telemetry in the clinical setting. Herzschrittmacherther Elektrophysiol. 2008;19(3):146–64.
31. SuperECG HeartBug product information. http://www.superecg.com/
32. Corventis company's NUVANT Mobile Cardiac Telemetry (MCT) System product information. http://www.corventis.com
33. AliveCor Heart Monitor product information. http://www.alivecor.com/
34. Razavi B. Design of analog CMOS integrated circuits. New York: Tata McGraw-Hill; 2002.

Chapter 2
System Architecture and Design Considerations

2.1 Wireless Capsule Endoscope

The wireless capsule endoscope system is a medical instrument, which can be used to visually examine the entire digestive tract wirelessly without any pain or risk associated with the conventional endoscopes. Unlike the conventional endoscopes manipulated using cables, the battery-operated wireless capsule endoscope is developed to transfer the image data using the RF transmission such as to avoid the pain and irritation to the digestive tract, which can be caused by the cables when using the conventional endoscopes. The first commercial capsule endoscope system [1] developed by Given Imaging has already been available in the market. Recently, research work on the capsule endoscope has been focusing on developing capsule endoscopes with enhanced image resolution, longer working time, and some extra functions [2–4].

The designed wireless capsule endoscope system is composed of a capsule, a portable data recorder, and an image workstation as shown in Fig. 2.1. The capsule inside the human body captures images and wirelessly transfers the data to the portable data recorder outside the body. In addition to the data recording function, the data recorder can serve as a bridge between the capsule and the workstation so that doctors can perform the real-time monitoring when data recorder is connected to the workstation using an USB connector. Control commands from the workstation can also be sent to the capsule through the data recorder, with a dedicated bidirectional communication protocol implemented in the system. Functionally, the designed wireless capsule endoscope is mainly composed of five major function blocks: a CMOS image sensor, an RF transceiver, a processing and controlling, the illumination LEDs, and the batteries. A commercial VGA image sensor has been adopted to provide 8-bit raw color filter array (CFA) images at a frame rate of 30 fps. The sensor consumes 40 mW in the active mode and less than 10 μA in the standby mode.

The work flow of the endoscope system is as follows. Once activated by the wake-up subsystem, the capsule circuit starts to work. First, the power management unit (PMU) converts 3 V battery voltage to the desired supply voltages for the other function blocks.

Z. Wang et al., *CMOS IC Design for Wireless Medical and Health Care*,
DOI 10.1007/978-1-4614-9503-1_2, © Springer Science+Business Media New York 2014

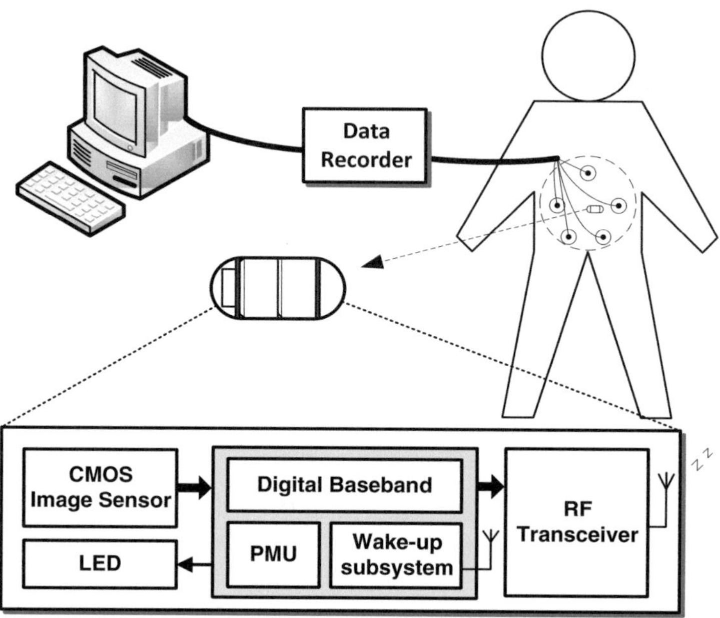

Fig. 2.1 Wireless capsule endoscope system

The on-chip oscillator generates clock signals for the digital baseband processing unit. The bidirectional communication link with the data recorder is established. With the control of baseband processing unit, a frame of image is captured, compressed, and transferred to the data recorder afterwards. At the end of the transmission of each image frame, the data recorder can send control commands to change the capsule working status such as the power mode and the image size. Once any exceptional situation is encountered, such as the interruption of communication link or the drop of battery voltage, the system would automatically enter the standby mode to save power and return to the normal mode periodically to listen to the communication link.

The main design challenges lies on the miniature-sized capsule. First, the battery-operated capsule is power-constrained strictly, and effective low-power techniques need to be employed to ensure adequately long working time. Second, the miniaturization requirement of the system leads to a strict constraint on the size of the printed circuit board (PCB) used for the capsule, and the circuits in the capsule should be highly integrated and the number of off-chip components should be reduced as few as possible. Third, an untouched wake-up function needs to be implemented to turn on/off the circuits after being hermetically encapsulated within the package. The wake-up function should also comply with the miniaturization and low-power requirements. A dedicated low-power SoC has been developed to meet these challenges.

The major part of the design idea on the capsule endoscope is to minimize the overall energy dissipation of the capsule system. Measurement has shown that RF part consumes more than 60 % of the overall energy. Unfortunately, further power optimization of the RF circuit is difficult. Instead, a system-level low-power technology is proposed by introducing the image compression module in the digital baseband unit, which results in the considerable data amount reduction and the power consumption reduction from the RF part consequently. Since the image compression module consumes much less power compared to the RF part, the overall average power reduction can be achieved. Note that the image compression is a computationally complex process, and the introduced extra hardware cost and power consumption for the compression turns to be another issue for our design. The coding complexity and the proper hardware architecture to implement the compression algorithm need to be carefully evaluated in consideration of the power consumption and the die size.

Another design issue is the system miniaturization. The whole capsule circuit needs to be encapsulated in a miniature package, where the PCB area is very limited. That means very few on-board components can be placed. In order to save the PCB area, it is necessary to integrate the PMU with as few on-board components as possible. Moreover, the values of the on-board components, such as capacitors, should be small enough to ensure their availability in the micro surface mounted device (SMD) package. Additionally, an effective calibration method should be provided for the chip as the on-chip resistors and capacitors suffer from the process variation.

The capsule endoscope needs to be turned on/off after being hermetically encapsulated within the package. Traditionally, this is achieved by using a magnetism-stimulated dry reed switch [5]. However, there are several disadvantages with the dry reed switch. First, it occupies a considerable PCB area even with the smallest package available. Second, the capsule should be surrounded by a magnet to keep power off state, which brings too much trouble to the production, storage, and transportation. To overcome these disadvantages, a passive wireless wake-up subsystem with the merits of zero standby current, high rejection to noise and disturbance is proposed to replace the dry reed switch. The wake-up subsystem recovers energy from the received 915 MHz RF signal modulated by the identification code, and zero standby power is consumed. This passive wireless link can be used not only for activating or resetting the system but also for the calibration of PMU by sending the calibration codes through this RF link.

2.2   Wireless Ligament Balance Measuring System in Total Knee Arthroplasty

The total knee arthroplasty (TKA) is an operation which replaces the damaged knee joint with the artificial knee implant, whereas the total hip replacement (THR) is an operation which replaces the damaged hip joint. The number of TKA and THR surgeries is increasing each year, especially in the developing countries such as China. As the average age of the population goes higher, it is estimated that the number of total knee and hip replacement surgeries will hit 3.48 million by 2030 [6]. For example, in China, about 80 % elder people are suffering from joint diseases. Among the surgeries, TKA surgeries account for about 30–50 %. It can release patients with degenerative joint disease from severe pain and immobility due to osteoarthritis. There were about 70,000 cases of TKA reported in China in 2010, and as forecasted the number will increase at speed of 10–15 % per year. However, TKA implants will fail because of wear, loosening, misalignment, etc. Dislocation of the prostheses is one of the most frequent and common complications after TKA. As a result, revision surgery will be conducted, bringing more pain to the patients [7–9]. In many cases, revision surgery has proven to be more traumatic and less successful than the initial surgery. Therefore, it is critical to ensure the success of the first operation to avoid injury. It becomes more and more important to avoid loosening and to improve the success ratio of the surgery. Successful surgery requires precise placement of implants such that the function of the joint is optimized biomechanically and biologically. Typically, most of these prosthetic implants are expected to work for at least 20 years with a successful TKA.

Many efforts have been made for early loosening detection. By providing an objective and quantitative measurement of the forces acting within the knee, the research carried out on the TKA is to help the surgeon improve the accuracy of the ligament balancing procedure, leading to a potentially longer prosthesis lifetime. The proper alignment of knee mechanical axis and the balance of collateral ligaments are crucial surgically controllable factors to ensure the successful outcomes and long-term lifespan of knee implants [10–12]. The absence of any of these two factors leads to uneven load distribution between the two compartments of tibial bearing surface and, consequently, to accelerated polyethylene wear, which results in unsuccessful clinical outcomes [13]. According to the literatures, many devices have been used intraoperatively to quantify the ligament balance [14–20]. These devices were only able to measure biomechanical parameters such as the extension gap [14], compressive tibiofemoral load [15], and bearing contact pressure [16, 17]. Furthermore, several shortcomings have been revealed in these devices such as the insufficient accuracy and the need to evert the patella during the measurement. Crottet et al. [18] have developed a force sensing device for intraoperative ligament balancing. The device consists of a sensitive plate on each condyle and a tibial base plate. The instrument is tested by a surgeon with a cadaver experiment. Wasielewski et al. [19, 20] used a pressure mapping system from Novel and attached it to the proximal surface of the tibial trials component with silicone adhesive. It was used intraoperatively for soft tissue balancing. The sensor map is connected to a data acquisition system, and the force and the pressure profiles are shown on a computer monitor.

In general, application-specific integrated circuits (ASIC) have the features of small size, low power, flexible functionality, and long-term reliability, which make them attractive for biomedical instrumentations [21]. A number of groups have incorporated electronic circuits in biomedical instrumentation and most of the research focus on monitoring the biomechanical implants or excessive wear and fatigue for preventing premature failures and for significantly reducing patient discomfort and risk [21–28]. Embedded implant sensors could provide new in vivo diagnostic capabilities that reduce these clinical complications and lead to improved implant materials and designs [25, 27]. In [23], in vivo strain gauges have been used in distal femoral replacements and in hip implants. However, in most of these experiments, the focus has been for logging data during short duration, and power is typically derived through inductive or ultrasonic coupling or through external leads in skin. In [19], temporary implants containing four load cells were used to harvest power and to measure knee joint forces.

The authors in [28] utilized an ASIC chip and other commercially available components to realize the instrument functions. The instrument is mainly used in dental prosthesis. The power consumption is 1.73 mW for 18 channels and the sampling frequency is only 111 Hz. In [21], an analog signal processing integrated circuit for microcantilever array has been designed for pressure measurement in biomedical applications. The chip consists of analog multiplexer, instrumentation amplifier, sample-and-hold circuit, on-chip voltage and current references, successive approximation register analog-to-digital converter (ADC), and digital control unit. The integrated circuit has been fabricated in 0.35 μm CMOS. In [29], an "active" acoustic method is presented. The acoustic waves are generated, e.g., by a mechanical hammer placed on the inside of the femoral hip stem wall. The mechanical-acoustic properties of the bone–implant interface give information about the status of the loosening process. A functional in vitro model of the measuring principle shows significant differences in varied phases of fixation. In [30], the authors describe an implantable system for the in vivo measurement of both micromotion and migration in THR and TKA. The system is based on a modified linear variable differential transformer (LVDT) whose null point is set automatically by a self-calibration algorithm. In [31], a finite element model was developed to predict the impingement and dislocation behavior of the prosthetic joint, for different combinations of cup orientation and patient maneuver. In [32], the authors develop a sensor- and sampling-based motion planner to control a surgical robot in order to explore osteolytic lesions in orthopedic surgery. The proposed method achieves 83–92 % performance rate when compared to methods that require 3D models of osteolytic cavities.

Although there are many methods to monitor the migration or loosening such as imaging techniques named Roentgen Stereophotogrammetric Analysis (RSA) [33], implantable system for in vivo measurement [30, 32], and some software for planning implantation and reimplantation interventions of hip joints [31, 34], most of them are just experimental ideas with no realistic data or preoperative planning, no in vivo measurement during the surgery. Moreover, the implanted electronic devices occupy space inside the femur. As a result, more bone should be removed to place them. In this book, a low-power system is designed to measure the position and pose of implants during the surgery and transmit the data wirelessly in vivo and display in 3D image. The system helps surgeons to make a precision judgment of the place of the implant during the surgery to avoid loosening or disjointing after surgery. The system will be used during the TKA operation which is the fundamental difference with [25]. Besides, this system has realized wireless data transmission which is different with other papers.

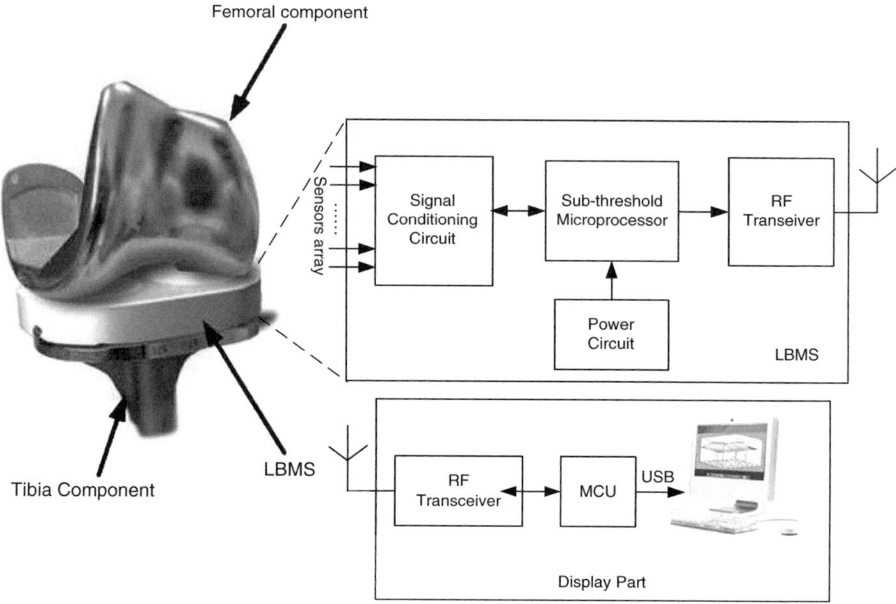

Fig. 2.2 System architecture of wireless ligament balance measuring in TKA

The architecture of the designed wireless ligament measuring system for TKA shown in Fig.2.2 consists of two parts: the Ligament Balance Measurement System (LBMS) and the display part. The LBMS is designed to measure the force and force distribution on the LBMS applied by the femoral component of the artificial implants and to transmit the force data wirelessly by a low-power transceiver. The LBMS composes of a sensors array (eight precise force sensors used in current system), an ultra-low-power microprocessor, and a low-power transceiver. The sensor array is formed by the pressure sensors of FSS series from Honeywell. The display part demonstrates the force data and its distribution in vivo in 3D images. The two parts of the system communicate with each other by the RF signal of 433 MHz. The RF transceiver working at the 400 MHz UHF band, with a 3 Mbps MSK transmitter and a 64 kbps OOK receiver, enables the feature of bidirectional communication between the LBMS and the external data logger. The MSK transmitter consumes only 3.9 mW power in total [35].

2.3   General System Architecture

From the two application examples above and some other existing wireless medical/ health care applications [36, 37], it can be observed that a typical wireless medical/ health care system is composed of the remote side and the local side as shown in Fig. 2.3. The data service center, the hospitals, and the doctors are at the remote side.

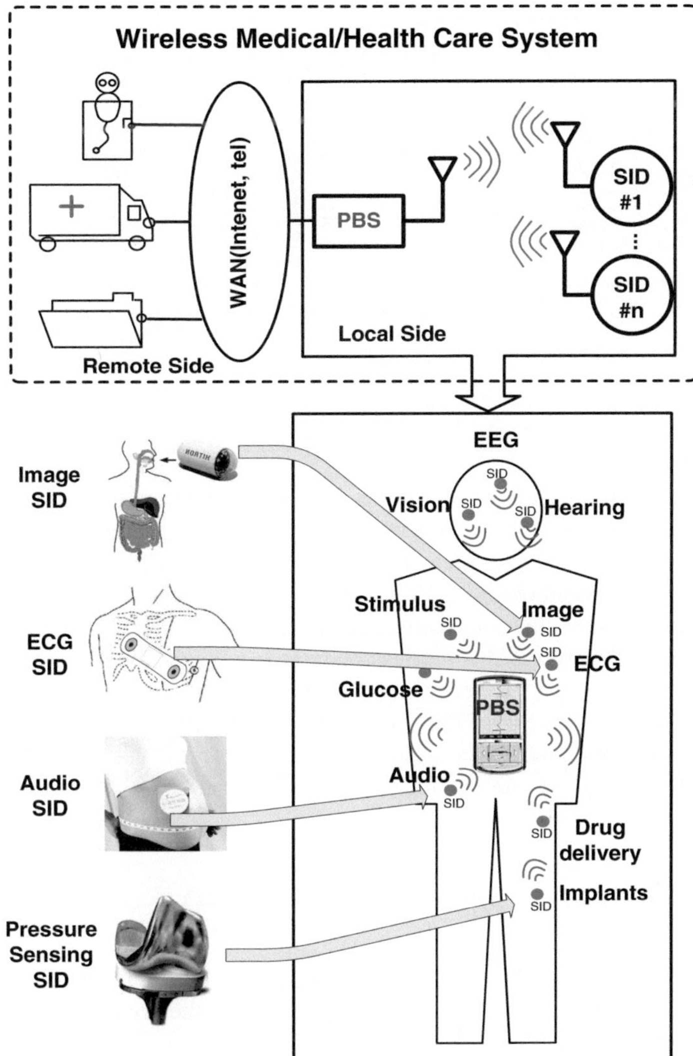

Fig. 2.3 System architecture of the wireless medical and health care applications

The remote side provides data storage, analysis, diagnosis, and other services. The local side refers to the equipment carried by the users. The local side is usually composed of one/multiple sensing/intervention devices (SIDs) and a portable base station (PBS).

The SIDs are attached to the human bodies directly, and they can be wearable or sometimes implantable. The most important function of SIDs is to sense/detect human vital signs and other physiological signals such as body temperature, blood pressure, blood glucose level, electrocardiograph (ECG) signals, etc. SIDs with

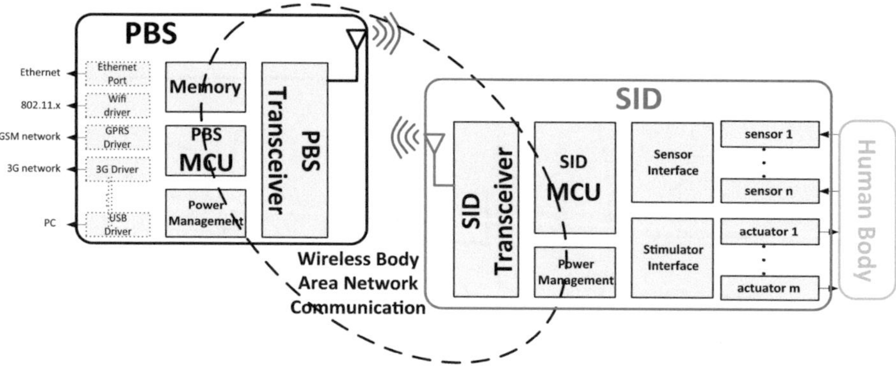

Fig. 2.4 PBS and SID in a wireless medical/health care system

advanced functions may have the ability to provide intervention stimulus to the human bodies. For example, an epilepsy control SID can promptly deliver drugs to the patient when the epilepsy presymptom is detected through continuous electro-encephalogram (EEG) monitoring. The PBS can be a specifically designed portable device, or just a mobile handset with some extra add-in functions. The PBS is connected to the SIDs through the wireless body area network (WBAN) communication. The PBS can be used to receive physiological data from the SIDs and to send control commands to the SIDs. The PBS is finally connected to remote side, namely, the hospital, doctors, ambulances, and data service centers via the wide area network (WAN) such as the internet and the mobile internet.

2.4   Design Considerations for PBS and SID

The detailed function blocks of the PBS and the SID at the local side in the wireless medical/health care system is shown in Fig. 2.4. And the content of this book is limited to the local side circuit design.

Note that the PBS mainly performs two functions, one is to communicate to the SIDs wirelessly, and the other is to connect to the WAN. As shown in Fig. 2.4, the PBS is usually composed of an MCU for system control, a PMU, a memory section for program/data storage, a transceiver to communicate with the SIDs, and the interface to Ethernet, WiFi, GPRS, etc., and the series port such as the USB port to PC and/or other devices.

A SID, as shown in the right part of Fig. 2.4, is usually composed of a light-weight MCU, an integrated PMU, and most importantly, the interfaces to biomedical sensors and biostimulators. The transceivers between the PBS and SIDs carry out the WBAN communication. In many situations, the PBS works with a set of SIDs for one personnel and a half-duplex single-hop star topology can be adopted [38].

From the viewpoint of implementation, the most critical constraint for SIDs is the device size. Since SIDs are usually powered by tiny coin batteries, the key point

Table 2.1 Comparison between PBS transceiver and SID transceiver

	PBS transceiver	SID transceiver
TRX frequency band	Multiband, cover 400/900/2,400 MHz ISM bands	Single band for one specific application
TRX data rate	10 kbps to 3 Mbps, reconfigurable	Fixed
TRX modulation	ASK, 2FSK, QPSK, MSK, changeable	Fixed
Power consumption	Moderately low	Ultra low

for SID circuit design is ultra-low-power (ULP) consumption. Every part of an SID has to be ULP, including the sensor interface, stimulator interface, flow controller, and the transceiver. All the circuit parts should be optimized in terms of power consumption, according to the specific application.

On the other hand, the PBS is usually powered by rechargeable Li-ion batteries, and the power limitation is not quite critical. Note that the SIDs are normally disposable, whereas the PBS should work with various SIDs and WAN connection with different communication speed, etc. Therefore, the most important challenge for PBS circuit design is its compatibility, both to the SIDs and the WAN.

One possible solution for the wireless medical/health care system is to build a powerful PBS transceiver with the highest compatibility and a set of dedicated SID SoCs optimized for different application purposes.

A multiband multimode PBS transceiver, which supports the body area wireless communication covering the 400 MHz/2.4 GHz ISM band, has been proposed, and the transceiver speed and modulation type is programmable to cover different data rate speed requirement for different SIDs. The power consumption imposed on the PBS SoC is not critical.

To work with this PBS SoC, application-optimized SID SoCs for different applications should be designed, such as ECG, pulse rate, EEG, and temperature monitoring. A SID SoC will only choose one frequency band and has fixed data rate and modulation type. The MCU program of an SID SoC can be fixed. The most important measure for an SID SoC is just the ULP consumption. The comparison between the PBS transceiver and the SID transceiver is shown in Table 2.1.

2.5   Choices of PBS and WBAN Transceivers

The WBAN transceiver is the most power-hungry part for the SIDs. To design a power efficient wireless medical/health care system, special attention should be paid to the WBAN transceiver selection. Since the other half the WBAN subsystem is inside the PBS, the PBS should also be taken into consideration.

Actually, there can be three choices for the PBS and WBAN transceivers and are as follows:

1. The first choice is to use a standard handset, such as a smartphone or tablet computer as the PBS, and use the standard-protocol short-range communication transceivers as the WBAN transceivers. Usually, a smartphone or tablet computer provides

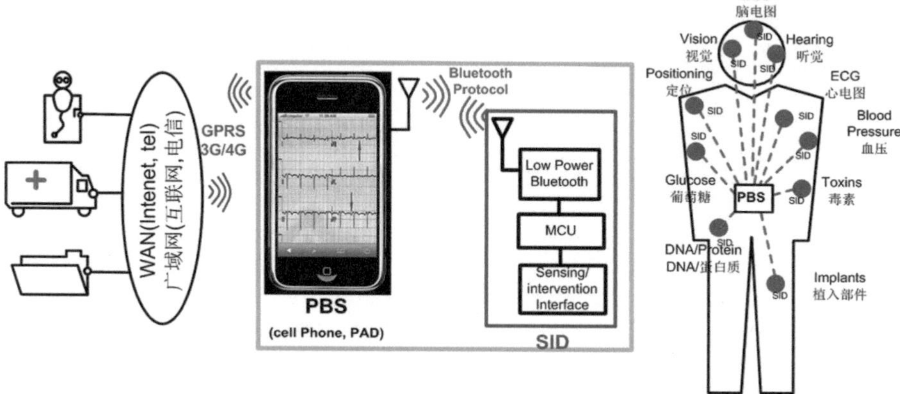

Fig. 2.5 A standard handset as PBS and standard-protocol for WBAN transceivers

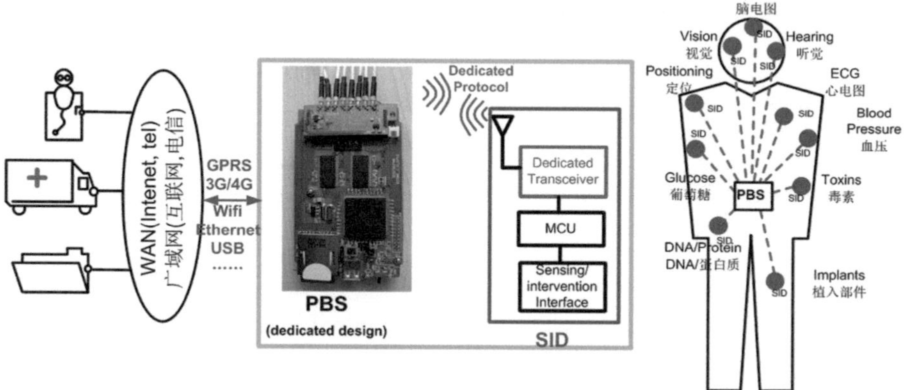

Fig. 2.6 A fully customized PBS with a dedicated protocol for WBAN transceivers

the short range connection via Bluetooth transceivers for low data rate transmission, and/or the WiFi transceivers for high data rate transmission as shown in Fig. 2.5. To comply with this system configuration, the SID should also have a standard-protocol transceiver.

The benefit of this section is that no hardware design is required for the PBS so that the product ramp-to-market time can be greatly saved. The shortcomings of this selection are also obvious. The SID has to use a standard-protocol transceiver, which is usually a stand-alone chip and is not quite power efficient. This will not be an optimal choice to implement an SID with stringent form factor and battery life requirement.

2. The second choice is to design a dedicated-protocol WBAN transceiver pair for the wireless medical/health care application system and to design a fully customized PBS as shown in Fig. 2.6 such as the system in [36].

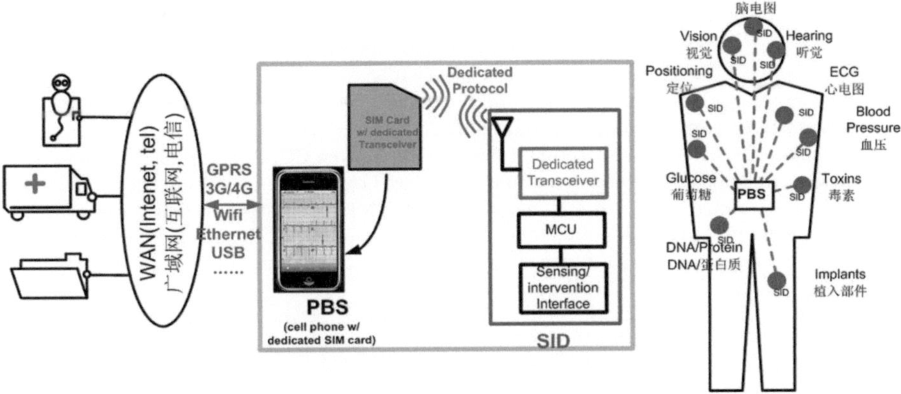

Fig. 2.7 A PBS using a standard handset with a dedicated protocol for WBAN transceivers

The major purpose of this method is to have a power-efficient transceiver for the SID. The drawback is that entire system design will be quite complicated, and the design cycle might be very long. Another drawback is the user has to carry an extra portable device (the PBS), and the user experience might not be good.

3. The third choice is still to design a dedicated-protocol WBAN transceiver pair. Compared to the second choice, the difference in this configuration is that a standard handset will be used as the PBS. The dedicated WBAN transceiver will be integrated in the handset accessories, such as the smartphone case, the memory card, and the SIM card as shown in Fig. 2.7. The ECG acquisition system in [37] is a good example, in which the ECG acquisition and the WBAN transceiver are both integrated in the smartphone case.

This configuration has the combined benefits of the previous two choices. The SID power efficiency can be optimized with a dedicated WBAN protocol, whereas there is no hardware design for the PBS, and the user can use the internet/mobile internet connection built inside the standard handset for WAN connections.

When building a practical wireless medical/health care application system, the designers need to make the optimal choice with a careful compromise among the system performance, such as SID size, SID power consumption, system complexity, design cycle, etc.

References

1. Iddan G, Meron G, Glukhovsky A, et al. Wireless capsule endoscopy. Nature. 2000;405: 417–8.
2. Park HJ, Ham HW, Song BS, et al. Design of bi-directional and multi-channel miniaturized telemetry module for wireless endoscopy. In: Proceedings of the 2nd annual international

IEEE-EMB special topic conference on microtechnologies in medicine and biology, Madison, WI, 2002. p. 273–6.

3. RF System Lab. [Online]. http://www.rfsystemlab.com

4. Xie X, Li G, Chen X, et al. A novel low power IC design for bi-directional digital wireless endoscopy capsule system. In: Proceedings of the IEEE international workshop on biomedical circuits and systems (BioCAS04), Singapore, 2004. p. S1.8.5–8.8.

5. Ginsberg GG, Barkun AN, Bosco JJ, Isenberg GA, Nguyen CC, Petersen BT, Silverman WB, Slivka A, Taitelbaum G. Wireless capsule endoscopy. Gastrointest Endosc. 2002;56(5):621–4.

6. Kurtz S. Total knee and hip replacement surgery projections show meteoric rise by 2030. Orthopaedic procedures set to continue gaining widespread acceptance as means to restore quality-of-life. In: Annual meeting of the American Academy of Orthopaedic Surgery, Mar 2006.

7. Platt SR, Farritor S, Haider H. On low-frequency electric power generation with PZT ceramics. ITTT ASME Trans Mechatron. 2005;10(2):240–52.

8. Chen H, Jia C, Chen Y, Liu M, Zhang C, Wang Z. A low-power ic design for the wireless monitoring system of the orthopedic implants. In: Proceedings of the 2008 custom integrated circuits conference (CICC2008), San Jose, CA, 21–24 Sept 2008, p. 363–6.

9. Almouahed S, Gouriou M, Hamitouche C, Stindel E, Roux C. Design and evaluation of instrumented smart knee implant. IEEE Trans Biomed Eng. 2011;58(4):971–82.

10. Insall JN, Binazzi R, Soudry M, Mestriner LA. Total knee arthroplasty. Clin Orthop Relat Res. 1985;192:13–22.

11. Dorr LD, Boiardo RA. Technical considerations in total knee arthroplasty. Clin Orthop Relat Res. 1986;205:5–11.

12. Wasielewski RC, Komistek RD. Computer-assisted ligament balancing of the femoral tibial joint using pressure sensors. In: Stiehl JB, Konermann WH, Haaker RG, DiGioia AM, editors. Navigation and MIS in orthopedic surgery, Berlin: Springer; 2007, Ch. 23. p. 175–81.

13. Viskontas DG, Skrinskas TV, Johnson JA, King GJ, Winemaker MJ, Chess DG. Computer-assisted gap equalization in total knee arthroplasty. J Arthroplasty. 2007;22(3):334–42.

14. Winemaker MJ. Perfect balance in total knee arthroplasty: the elusive compromise. J Arthroplasty. 2002;17(1):2–10.

15. Morris BA, D'Lima DD, Slamin J, Kovacevic N, Arms SW, Townsend CP, Colwell Jr CW. e-knee: evolution of the electronic knee prosthesis - telemetry technology development. J Bone Joint Surg. 2001;83-A:62–6.

16. Takahashi T, Wada Y, Yamamoto H. Soft-tissue balancing with pressure distribution during total knee arthroplasty. J Bone Joint Surg. 1997;79(2):235–9.

17. Wallace AL, Harris ML, Walsh WR, Bruce WJM. Intraoperative assessment of tibiofemoral contact stresses in total knee arthroplasty. J Arthroplasty. 1998;13(8):923–7.

18. Crottet D, Maeder T, Fritschy D, Bleuler H, Nolte L-P, Pappas IP. Development of a force amplitude-and-location-sensing device designed to improve the ligament balancing procedure in TKA. IEEE Trans Biomed Eng. 2005;52:1609–11.

19. Wasielewski RC, Galat DD, Komistek RD. An intraoperative pressure-measuring device used in total knee arthoplasties and its kinematics correlations. Clin Orthop Rel Res. 2004;(427):171–8.

20. Wasielewski RC, Galat DD, Komistek RD. Correlation of compartment pressure data from an intraoperative sensing device with postoperative fluoroscopic kinematic results in TKA patients. J Biomech. 2005;38:333–9.

21. Qu W, Islam SK, Mahfouz MR, Haider MR, To G, Mostafa S, et al. Microcantilever array pressure measurement system for biomedical instrumentation. IEEE Sens J. 2010;10(2):321–30.

22. Le TT, Han J, von Jouanne A, et al. Piezoelectric micro-power generation interface circuits. IEEE J Solid-State Circuits. 2006;41(6):1411–20.

23. Taylor SJG, Walker PS. Forces and moments telemetered from two distal femoral replacements during various activities. J Biomech. 2001;34:839–48.

24. Gerrish P, Herrmann E, Tyler L, Walsh K. Challenges and constraints in designing implantable medical ICs. IEEE Trans Dev Mater Reliab. 2005;5(3):435–44.

25. Chen H, Liu M, Hao W, Chen Y, Zhang C, Wang Z. Low-power circuits for the bidirectional wireless monitoring system of the orthopedic implants. IEEE Trans Biomed Circuits Syst. 2009;3(6):437–43.
26. Chen H, Liu M, Jia C, Wang Z. Power harvesting using PZT ceramics in orthopedic implants. IEEE Trans Ultrason Ferroelectr Freq Control. 2009;56(9):2010–4.
27. Ottman GK, Hofmann HF, Lesieutre GA. A piezo-powered floating-gate sensor array for long-term fatigue monitoring in biomechanical implants. IEEE Trans Biomed Circuits Syst. 2008;2(3):164–72.
28. Claes W, Sansen W, Puers R. A 40µA/channel compensated 18-channel strain gauge measurement system for stress monitoring in dental implants. IEEE J Solid-State Circuits. 2002; 37:293–301.
29. Ewald H, Ruther C, Mittelmeier W, Bader R, Kluess D. A novel in vivo sensor for loosening diagnostics in total hip replacement. In: 2011 IEEE sensors, 28–31 Oct 2011. p. 89–92.
30. Hao S, Taylor J, Miles AW, Bowen CR. An implantable system for the in vivo measure measurement of hip and knee migration and micromotion. In: International conference on signals and electronic systems, Kraków, 14–17 Sept 2008. p. 445–8.
31. Ghaffari M, Nickmanesh R, Tamannaee N, Farahmand F. The impingement-dislocation risk of total hip replacement: effects of cup orientation and patient maneuvers. In: 34th annual international conference of the IEEE EMBS, San Diego, CA, 28 Aug–1 Sept 2012. p.6801–4.
32. Liu WP, Lucas BC, Guerin K, Plaku E. Sensor and sampling-based motion planning for minimally invasive robotic exploration of osteolytic lesions. In: 2011 IEEE/RSJ international conference on intelligent robots and systems, San Francisco, CA, 25–30 Sept 2011. p. 1346–52.
33. Selvik G. Roentgen stereophotogrammetric analysis. Acta Radiol. 1990;31:113–26.
34. Michalikova M, Bednarcikova L, Petrik M, Rasi R, Zivcak J. The digital pre-operative planning of total hip replacements. In: IEEE 8th international symposium on applied machine intelligence and informatics (SAMI), Herl'any, Slovakia, 28–30 Jan 2010, p. 279–82.
35. Jiang H, Li F, Chen X, Ning Y, Zhang X, Zhang B, Ma T, Wang Z. A SoC with 3.9mW 3Mbps UHF transmitter and 240µW MCU for capsule endoscope with bidirectional communication. In: 2010 IEEE Asian solid state circuits conference (A-SSCC), Beijing, 8–10 Nov 2010. p. 1–4(9-3).
36. Corventis company's NUVANT Mobile Cardiac Telemetry (MCT) System product information. http://www.corventis.com
37. AliveCor Heart Monitor product information. http://www.alivecor.com/
38. Yang GZ. Body sensor networks. London: Springer; 2006.

Chapter 3
Biomedical Signal Acquisition Circuits

3.1 Biomedical Sensors

The biomedical sensor is one of the most significant parts in a wireless medical/ health care system. Various types of biomedical sensors are used to acquire the human body information. A modern biomedical sensor is usually a digital sensor, which means the final output of the sensor is a digital electrical signal. A typical digital biomedical sensor is composed of a transducer for signal energy conversion, an interface circuit to buffer the transducer output, and a digitizer to digitize the signal as shown in Fig. 3.1. The interface circuit and the digitizer circuit forms the sensor readout circuit and can usually be implemented within one integrated circuit using the CMOS technologies.

In the biomedical sensor, the transducer first converts the body information signal in one form of energy to another form of energy, namely, an electrical signal. The original energy types include mechanical, chemical, optical, magnetic, thermal, acoustic, electrical, and some other types of energy.

1. Mechanical signals, such as force, pressure, torque, capacity, thickness, mass, position, velocity, acceleration, angle, loudness, etc. A typical type of mechanical sensor is the force sensor, such as the FSS-SMT series low-profile force sensor [1] manufactured by Honeywell as shown in Fig. 3.2, which can be used to measure the pressure inside a human organ or joint.
2. Chemical signals, such as pH, saturation, solubility, protein, reaction speed, enzyme, oxidation–reduction, etc. One commonly seen chemical sensor is the pH sensor, which can be used to build a capsule to identify the presence of acid reflux caused by caused by gastroesophageal reflux disease (GERD) [2], such as the Bravo® pH monitoring system as shown in Fig. 3.3, which is now manufactured by Given Imaging.
3. Optical signals, such as intensity, luminance, wavelength, polarization, phase, reflectivity, refractivity, etc. The widely used image sensor is one typical optical sensor.

Z. Wang et al., *CMOS IC Design for Wireless Medical and Health Care*,
DOI 10.1007/978-1-4614-9503-1_3, © Springer Science+Business Media New York 2014

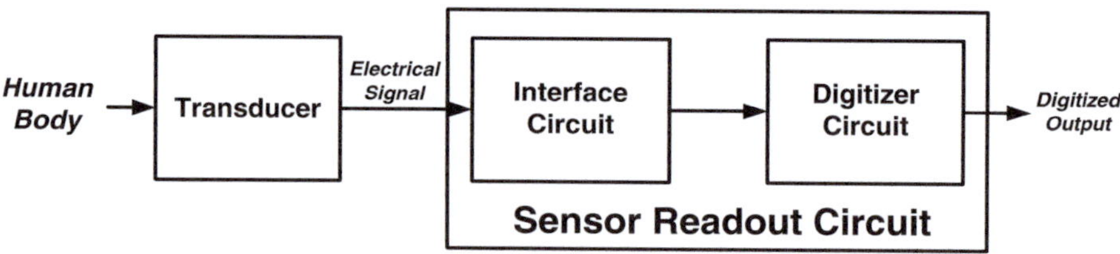

Fig. 3.1 Block diagram of a digital biomedical sensor

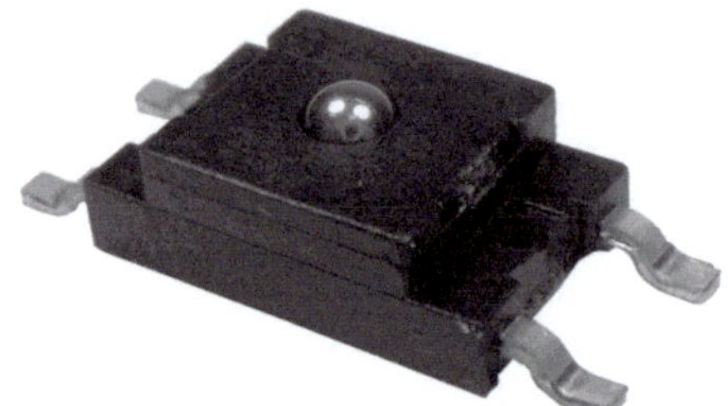

Fig. 3.2 Honeywell
low-profile force sensor
(package size
13.7 mm×5.6 mm×3.76 mm,
including soldering pins) [1]

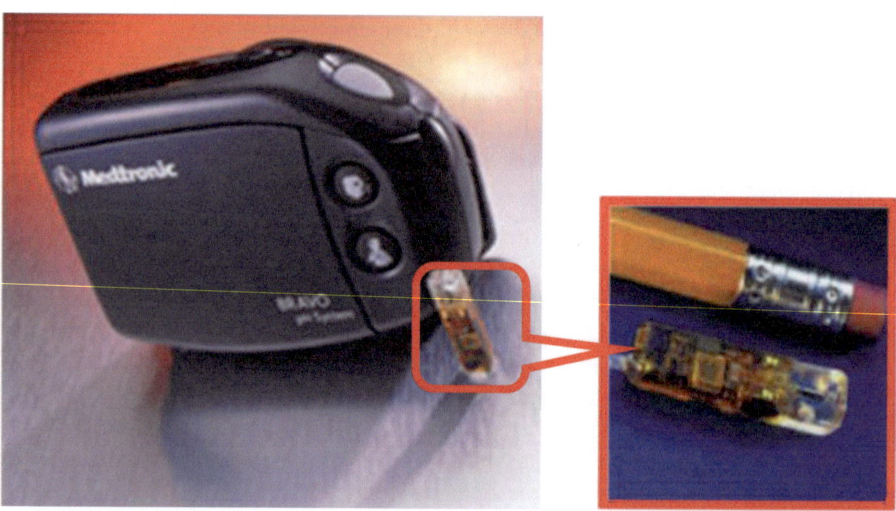

Fig. 3.3 Bravo® pH monitoring system including the pH capsule the portable data receiver, originally manufactured by Medtronic, now acquired by Given Imaging. The pH capsule containing the pH sensor is shown on the right side. The pictures are available online http://www.digestivehealthcare. com/bravo_ph.html

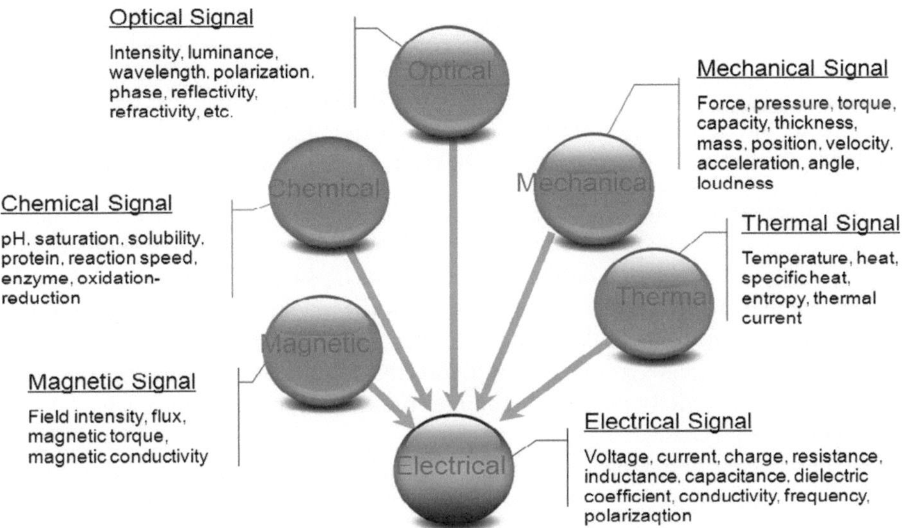

Fig. 3.4 Signal energy conversion by the transducer in a biomedical sensor

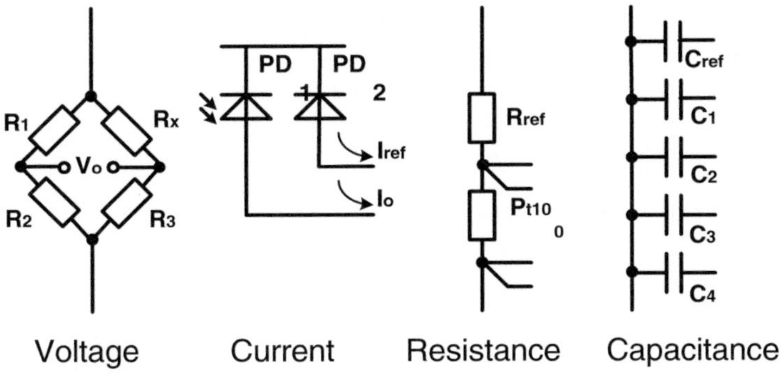

Fig. 3.5 Electrical signal types that can be handled by sensor circuits

4. Magnetic signals, such as field intensity, flux, magnetic torque, magnetic conductivity, etc. Nowadays, 3D miniature magnetic sensors for orientation detection can be easily found in the smartphones. These sensors can also find significant usage in the wireless medical and health care systems.
5. Thermal signals, such as temperature, heat, specific heat, entropy, thermal current, etc.

In a digital sensor, no matter what type of energy the original signal is, the transducer first converts the original signal energy into electrical signals that can be further handled by the interface circuit and the following digitizer as shown in Fig. 3.4. The typical electrical signal type can be voltage, current, resistance, capacitance, etc. as shown in Fig. 3.5. We will then need an interface circuit to buffer the electrical signal before sending it to the digitization circuit.

3.2   Sensor Interface Circuits

The sensor interface circuit is a bridge between the transducer and the digitizer. It converts the transducer's output signal into a signal that can be accepted by the digitizer. It can be used to perform one or multiple functions as listed below:

- Signal conversion: for example, to convert the resistance/capacitance value into a voltage or current signal that an analog-to-digital converter (ADC) can process.
- Signal amplification: the output signal from the transducer is usually quite weak, and a gain stage is usually required to match the input range of the digitizer. For instance, the peak-to-peak value of an electrocardiography (ECG) signal from the electrodes ranges from a few millivolts to several tens of millivolts [3]; a gain amplifier is definitely required to amplify the ECG signal first before the analog-to-digital conversion.
- Signal driving: the transducer usually has very limited driving capability, and it is quite difficult for a transducer to directly drive a digitizer with large input capacitance or small input resistance. The sensor interface circuit is then needed to enhance the signal driving capability.
- Other functions, such as impedance matching, dc voltage shifting, common-mode rejection, noise filtering, offset voltage cancelling, motion artifacts removing, etc.

The following part of this subsection provides two design examples to illustrate the design principles of biomedical sensor interface circuit.

3.2.1   Interface Circuit to Capacitive Sensors

Some biomedical sensors' output electrical signal is the capacitance, and an interface circuit is usually employed to convert the capacitance into a voltage signal.

The traditional interface circuit for capacitive sensors array is shown in Fig. 3.6a. This type interface with switched-capacitor amplifier structure is widely used for capacitance-to-voltage conversion or sample-and-hold operation with relatively high update rate [4].

In one conversion cycle, the measured capacitor C_X samples the reference voltage V_{REF} first, and then the charge of $V_{REF} \cdot C_X$ is injected into C_F to produce an output voltage as:

$$V_{SH} = -V_{REF} \cdot C_X / C_F \tag{3.1}$$

Assuming the reference voltage is $-V_{SS}$, and the maximum V_{SH} is from Gnd to V_{DD}. The measurement range is given as:

$$0 < C_X < C_F \tag{3.2}$$

Because the largest on-chip capacitor devices in modern semiconductor process are on the order of dozens of pF, the measurement range of traditional capacitive

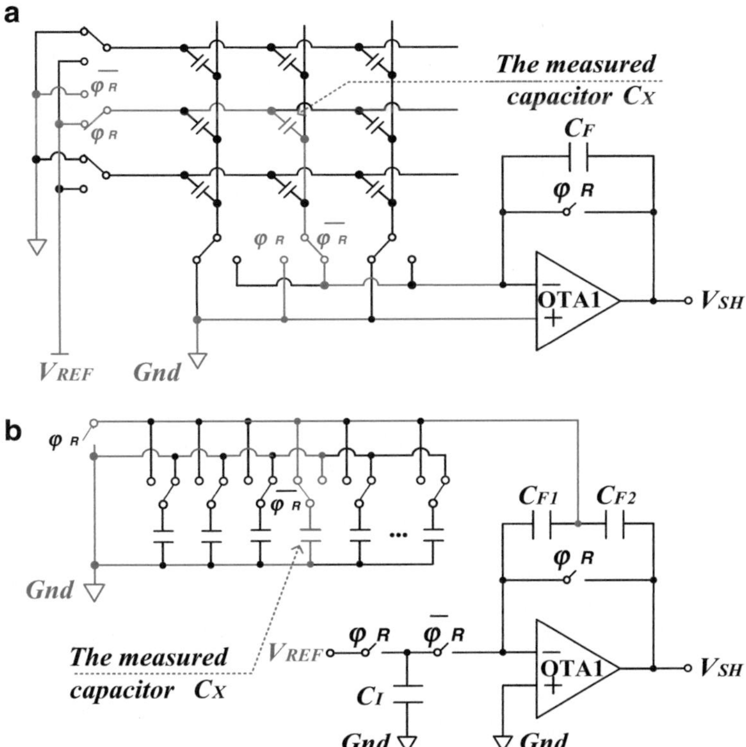

Fig. 3.6 Capacitance–voltage converter (CVC) for capacitive sensors array: (**a**) a traditional CVC, (**b**) a new CVC

interface is usually difficult to exceed this order. Even if an off-chip capacitor with higher capacitance could be used as C_F, the OTA should have a relatively high slew rate, leading to higher power consumption.

Of course, if a lower reference voltage V_{REF} is used in Fig. 3.6a, the capacitance measurement range could be enlarged. However, a precision voltage generator with high driving ability and low noise performance is required, which will inevitably increase the complexity of the system.

To obtain a wide capacitance measurement range with CMOS on-chip capacitor devices, a novel switched-capacitor amplifier structure with T-type feedback network can be used. As shown in Fig. 3.7b, the measured capacitor is set as a part of feedback network, which includes C_I, C_X, C_{F1} and C_{F2}. The measured capacitor C_X is selected from sensors array by 16-channel multiplexer and set as a part of the switched-capacitor feedback network. The ground of the sensors is denoted as Gnd.

In the reset phase of one conversion cycle as shown in Fig. 3.7a, C_I is first charged to V_{REF} and the other terminal voltages of capacitors are set to Gnd.

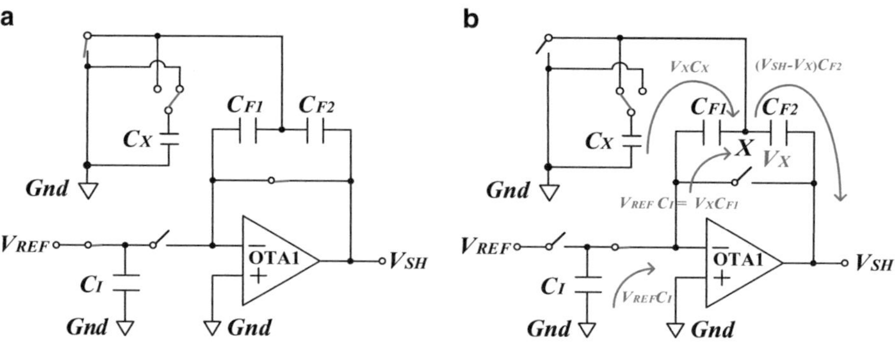

Fig. 3.7 Operation of new CVC: (**a**) reset phase, (**b**) conversion phase

In the conversion phase, a constant amount of charge $V_{REF} \cdot C_I$ is injected into C_{F1} to produce a middle-node voltage as:

$$V_X = -V_{REF} \cdot C_I / C_{F1} \tag{3.3}$$

The variations of V_X cause the charge redistribution between C_X and C_{F2}, which are $V_X C_X$ from *Gnd* to node X and $(V_{SH} - V_X)C_{F2}$ from node X to the output node. According to charge balancing on node X and assuming $C_{F1} = C_{F2} = C_F$, the sampled voltage on the output node is given as:

$$V_{SH} = -V_{REF} \cdot \left(2C_I / C_F + C_I \cdot C_X / C_F^2\right) \tag{3.4}$$

Since $0 < V_{SH} < V_{DD}$, the input capacitance range can be expressed as:

$$0 < C_X < C_F \left(C_F / C_I - 2\right) \tag{3.5}$$

V_{SH} is linearly proportional to the measured capacitance C_X. To obtain V_{SH}, the operational amplifier OTA1 charges C_{F2}, instead of directly charging C_X. As a result, only a little amount of charge needs to be injected into the measured capacitor C_X. The amount of charge transfer is only $V_{REF}(C_I + C_I C_X / C_F)$, which corresponds to $V_{REF} C_X$ of the described capacitance–voltage converter (CVC) with traditional structure. By setting $C_X >> C_F >> C_I$, this method can extend the CVC's input range and reduce the OTA's slew rate requirement obviously. Therefore, it does not need to design a special output stage for OTA. The new CVC reduces the structure complexity and the power consumption of OTA effectively. With the features of high update rate and low power consumption, the new CVC is quite suitable for interfacing of capacitive sensors array with wide capacitance measurement range.

The OTA noise transfer function is a key issue to the output noise. For noise analyzing, the equivalent model in Fig. 3.8 can be used. The sampled voltage V_{SH} at the output node of the traditional structure in Fig. 3.8a and the new structure in Fig. 3.8b can be, respectively, rewritten as:

$$V_{SH} = -V_{REF} C_X / C_F + \left(1 + C_X / C_F\right) \cdot V_{ni} \tag{3.6}$$

$$V_{SH} = -V_{REF} \left(2C_I / C_F + C_I C_X / C_F^2\right) + \left(1 + C_I / C_F\right)\left(2 + C_X / C_F\right) \cdot V_{ni} \tag{3.7}$$

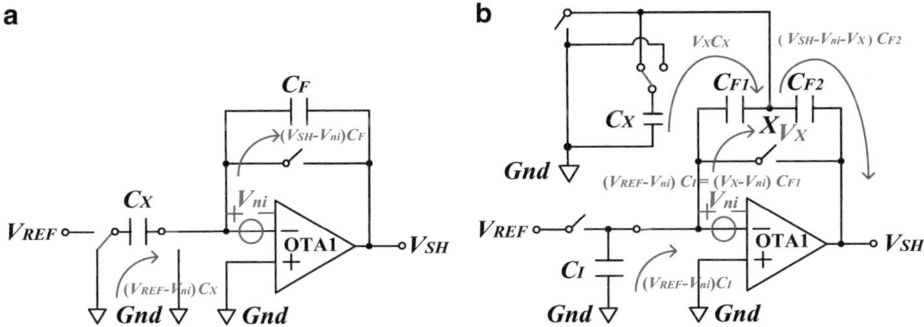

Fig. 3.8 Equivalent model for noise analyzing: (**a**) the traditional CVC, (**b**) the new CVC

where V_{ni} is the equivalent input noise of OTA. Because the new structure has a larger T-ratio C_X/C_F, the output noise from OTA in T-type network is larger than in conventional switched-capacitor network, which will degrade the input capacitance range of CVC. Thus, the ratio of C_X to C_F is also a tradeoff parameter in the T-network design. In the practical design, V_{REF} is connected to $-V_{SS}$, the value of C_I is set as 1 pF, and the capacitance of C_{F1} or C_{F2} is 20 pF, the measurement range of the new CVC can be from 0 pF (open circuit) to 360 pF theoretically. Due to the noise and the output nonlinearity of OTA, the maximum voltage on output node V_{SH} is difficult to reach V_{DD}. The practical linear input range of the presented CVC is about 350 pF with ±0.9 V power supply.

Additionally, the noise of the new CVC is also partially affected by the clock-through and charge injection of the switches, resulting in some redundant charges injected to the T-type capacitors network. In order to avoid affecting the dynamic range of the CVC, nonoverlapping clock and complementary switches can be utilized.

3.2.2   Instrument Amplifier for Voltage Sensor Interface

High-performance instrument amplifiers are widely used in voltage sensor interface circuits to measure microvolt level signals [5–11]. In order to amplify weak signals accurately, an IA is required to have low noise, low offset voltage, high input impedance, high common-mode rejection ratio (CMRR), and power supply rejection ratio (PSRR). It is also needed to have small area and low power consumption while is used in a portable, low cost, battery-powered wireless medical/health care system.

To implement the IAs using the CMOS technologies, design techniques should be used to overcome the problems associated with the CMOS technologies, such as the lower transconductance (g_m), higher noise, and worse matching [12], compared to the bipolar technologies. Techniques such as chopper and auto-zero are usually used to improve CMOS IA performance [13].

An IA can take use of either the resistive feedback structure [14] in which three operational amplifiers (op-amp) are used or the current feedback [15] configuration.

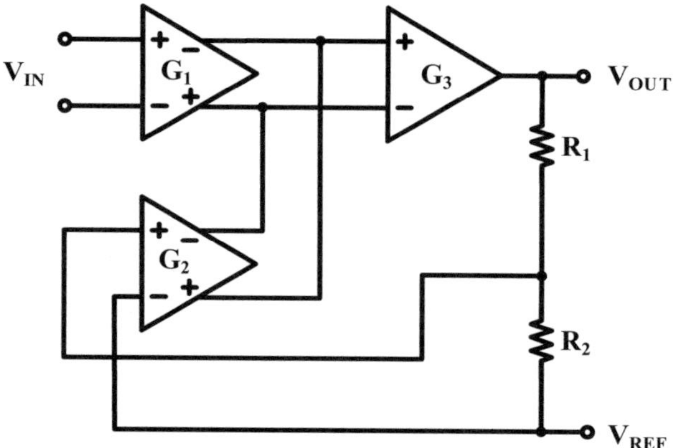

Fig. 3.9 The block diagram of a typical indirect current feedback IA

The latter one may have higher CMRR and wider bandwidth [16]. There are direct and indirect current feedback structures. The block diagram of a typical indirect current feedback IA is drawn in Fig. 3.9. The transconductance G_1 only transfers differential input signal to output current. The common input signal is thus isolated from the feedback loop and it hardly takes effect on the output signal. This type of IA has a low offset and a high efficiency. It is a good choice for the biomedical sensor interface circuit.

However, the offset of the first stage amplifier, which is between two modulators, will be modulated to the chopper frequency at final output and generates ripple. This ripple can be suppressed by a cascaded low pass filter at the cost of large area and high power consumption. Several techniques can be found in literature to reduce the ripple without using the external filter.

In [17], the first stage employs a chopper amplifier in a low-frequency path to cancel the offset of the wide-bandwidth amplifier. A sample-and-hold circuit is used to reduce the ripple. This is a feed-forward structure. So the circuit should be carefully designed considering process, voltage, and temperature variances. In [18], a switch capacitor (SC) notch filter is inserted to reduce ripple at chopper frequency. The switches in the SC circuit may induce extra charge injection and clock feed-through. A capacitive coupled chopper IA is proposed in [8]. The input capacitor removes the op-amp's offset. However, the input impedance is limited to tens of Mega Ohms even with impedance boost circuit. A more effect way to reduce the ripple is to use feedback. Kusuda [19, 20] propose a local feedback technique named as Auto Correction Feedback (ACFB) for a chopper amplifier to suppress its offset related ripple.

Most conventional techniques studied how to suppress ripple by taking different circuit structures. This subsection puts emphasis on analyzing the relationships between input signal and offset while they are processed in an amplifier. Then a new design method to amplify the signal and suppress the offset at the same time will be discussed. In this new technique, a bandpass amplifier is used as the first stage of the IA, and a ripple reduction loop (RRL) is also adopted such that output ripple is highly reduced.

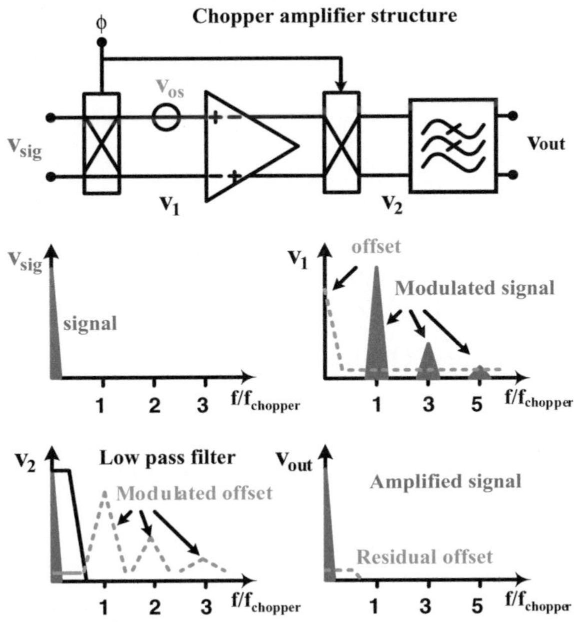

Fig. 3.10 Working principle of the chopper technique

Working Principle

Figure 3.10 describes the working principle of the chopper technique. The signal v_{sig} is modulated to chopper frequency $f_{chopper}$ before it is amplified so as to be separated with the input referred offset v_{os} of the amplifier in frequency domain. Then the signal is processed by the amplifier and modulated back.

The amplitude frequency response of the amplifier is drawn in Fig. 3.11. After the signal is modulated once to the chopper frequency, it is clear to see that v_{sig} has less gain than v_{os} has for the limit bandwidth (BW) of the amplifier. In other words, the output signal to offset ratio of the amplifier is smaller than the input signal to offset ratio. The ripple effect should then be taken careful consideration.

On way to alleviate the problem is to set the chopper frequency inside the BW as shown in Fig. 3.11a. However, the amplifier which is used in an IA as a feed forward path is always an op-amp with a large gain and a small BW. It needs to consume quite large power to enlarge its BW (also its gain bandwidth product, GBW) while processing signals with a high chopper frequency. On the other hand, if the chopper frequency is higher than the BW in Fig. 3.11b, the gain difference between v_{os} and v_{sig} will be larger.

In most situations, the amplifier can be composed of two or even more stages. A two-stage amplifier using the chopper technique is shown in Fig. 3.12. The chopper modulators before A1 and after A1 are controlled by the chopper clock φ. A typical two-stage amplifier, which consists of a folded cascode input stage, a common source output stage with Miller compensation capacitor C_C, is drawn in Fig. 3.13.

Three chopper switches may be added to the amplifier in Fig. 3.13 to form a chopper amplifier shown in Fig. 3.12, with one at the input node and the other two at the

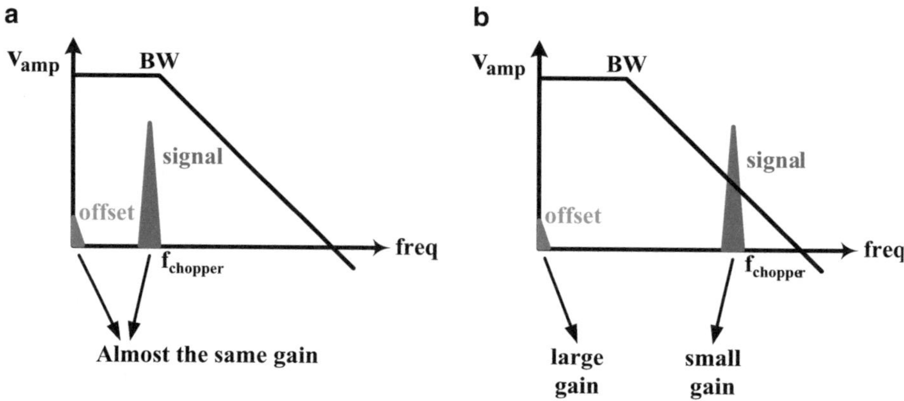

Fig. 3.11 The relationship between the chopper frequency and the amplifier's BW, (**a**) the chopper frequency is lower than the BW, (**b**) the chopper frequency is higher than the BW

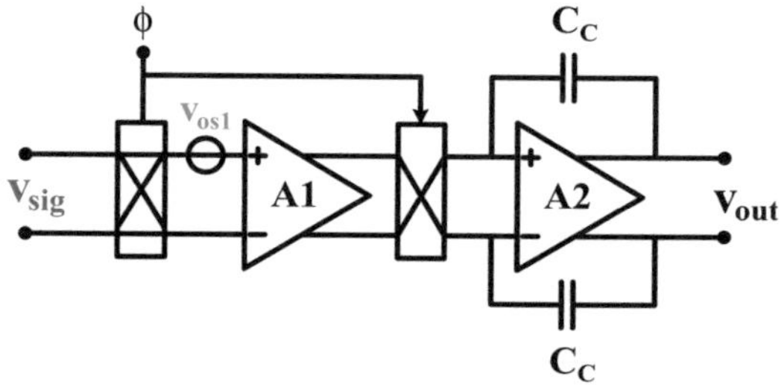

Fig. 3.12 A two-stage amplifier using the chopper technique

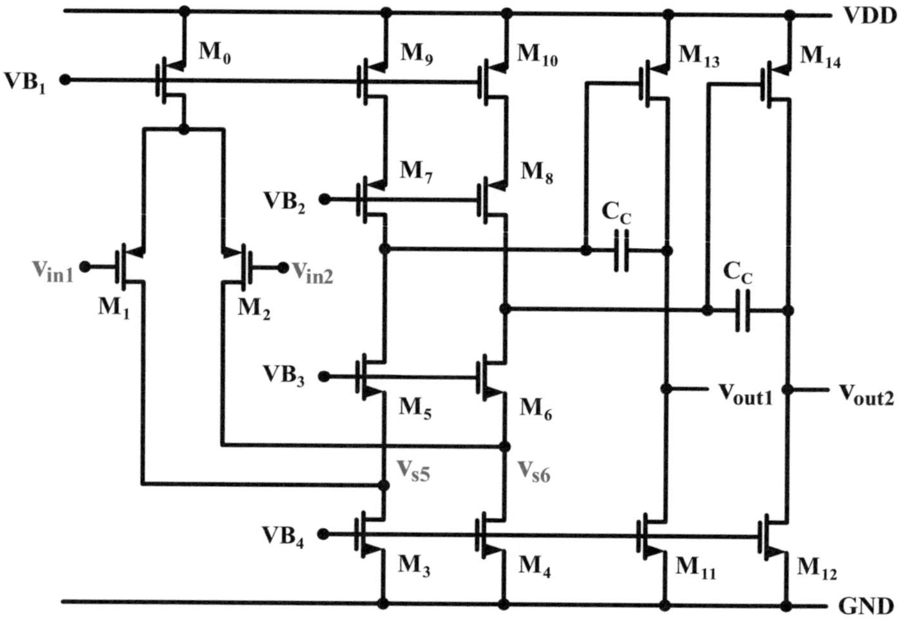

Fig. 3.13 A two-stage amplifier with Miller compensation

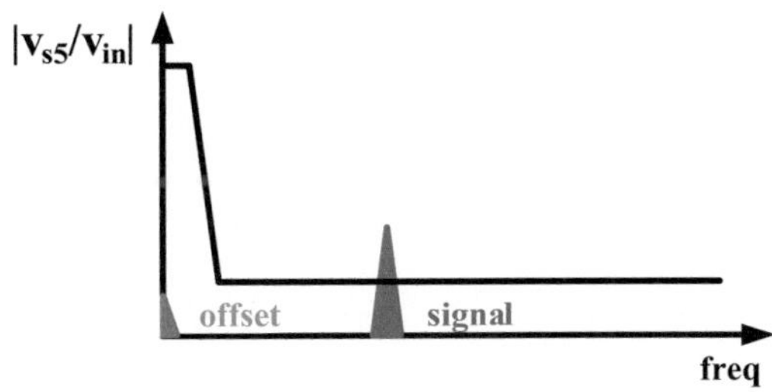

Fig. 3.14 Frequency response of each stage of a two-stage amplifier

source of cascode transistors [21]. The impedance seen from the source of transistor M_5 is written in (3.8), where g_{mx} and r_{ox} are the transconductance and the output resistance of transistor M_x, respectively. At low frequency, the Miller compensation capacitor C_C can be viewed as an open circuit. So the impedance is large as in (3.9). At high frequency, C_C is more like a short circuit and the impedance drops to $1/g_{m5}$ as shown in (3.10). As a result, the voltage gain from node voltage $v_{in1,2}$ to node voltage $v_{s5,6}$ is also large at the low frequency and then decreases with the frequency. The expressions are shown in (3.11) and (3.12), while the amplitude frequency response is drawn in Fig. 3.14. Obviously, the offset due to M1–M4 acquires larger gain than the input signal in this cascode stage. The analysis could be extended to similar circuits, such as the op-amp with a Miller capacitor in the indirect feedback IA.

$$
Z_{in\_M5} = \frac{\dfrac{\left[\left(g_{m7}r_{o7}\right)r_{o9} + r_{o7} + r_{o9}\right] // \dfrac{1}{sC_C}}{r_{o5}} + 1}{g_{m5}}
\tag{3.8}
$$

$$
\left|Z_{in\_M5}\right|_{at\_low\_frequency} \approx \frac{\dfrac{\left(g_{m7}r_{o7}\right)r_{o9} + r_{o7} + r_{o9}}{r_{o5}} + 1}{g_{m5}} \approx \frac{g_{m7}r_{o7}r_{o9}}{g_{m5}r_{o5}}
\tag{3.9}
$$

$$
\left|Z_{in\_M5}\right|_{at\_high\_frequency} \approx \left|\frac{\dfrac{1}{sr_{o5}C_C} + 1}{g_{m5}}\right| \approx \frac{1}{g_{m5}}
\tag{3.10}
$$

$$
\left|\frac{v_{s5}}{v_{in1}}\right|_{at\_low\_frequency} = g_{m1}\left(r_{o1} // r_{o3} // \frac{g_{m7}r_{o7}r_{o9}}{g_{m5}r_{o5}}\right)
\tag{3.11}
$$

$$
\left|\frac{v_{s5}}{v_{in1}}\right|_{at\_high\_frequency} = g_{m1}\left(r_{o1} // r_{o3} // \frac{1}{g_{m5}}\right) \approx \frac{g_{m1}}{g_{m5}}
\tag{3.12}
$$

A bandpass input stage can be used to suppress the offset and amplify the signal meanwhile. The center frequency of the pass band is selected at chopper frequency $f_{chopper}$. The ripple reduction effect of the bandpass amplifier is shown in Fig. 3.15.

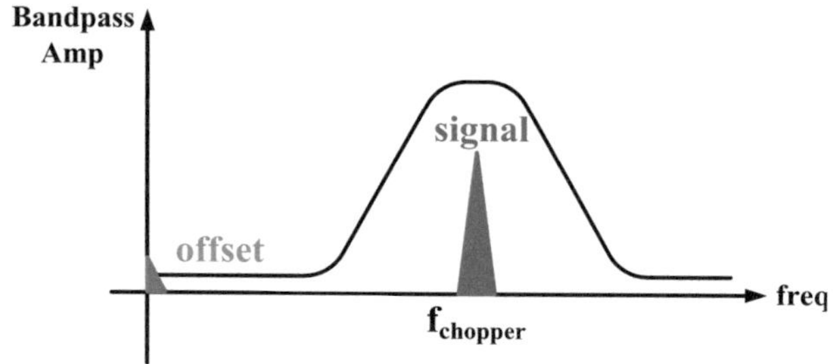

Fig. 3.15 Ripple reduction effect of the bandpass amplifier

This structure has several benefits. First, the offset caused by input transistors is suppressed instead of amplified. So the output ripple is also reduced. Second, the input transistors can be designed with small size so that the input impedance is increased. Third, the input signal has larger gain than in a traditional low pass amplifier while the chopper frequency is not limited by the BW. Fourth, the bandpass amplifier can be designed taking use of active inductors that occupy small area and consume little power.

A method to add a bandpass filter between the two chopper modulators is presented in [22] and [23]. It is mainly used to reduce the residual offset induced by the nonideal effects from the first chopper switches such as charge injection. A new structure similar to those structures will be discussed in this subsection. The main difference compared to the conventional structures is that this new structure uses a *bandpass amplifier* with active inductor load, whereas the conventional techniques use the *bandpass filter*. The new circuit technique to use a bandpass amplifier can both suppress the offset and reduce the residual offset, whereas the bandpass filter can only achieve the latter.

CMOS Circuit Realization

An indirect current feedback IA has high CMRR, high input impedance, and high efficiency. The block diagram of such an IA with a bandpass input stage is shown in Fig. 3.16. The input voltage signal and the feedback voltage signal are converted to currents through transconductance stages G_1 and G_2, respectively. These currents are added together and converted back to a voltage signal by the bandpass loads, which make use of active inductors. This voltage signal is further processed by the class AB output stage, which consists of G_3 and G_4. The RRL senses the voltage ripple at final output node and injects feedback currents to the inputs of the second modulator. The bandgap block generates reference voltages and currents for the whole circuit. The IA voltage gain is determined by the ratio of resistor R_1 and R_2 as shown in (3.13), if G_1 and G_2 have the same transconductance value.

$$G_{IA} = \frac{2R_1 + R_2}{R_2} \qquad (3.13)$$

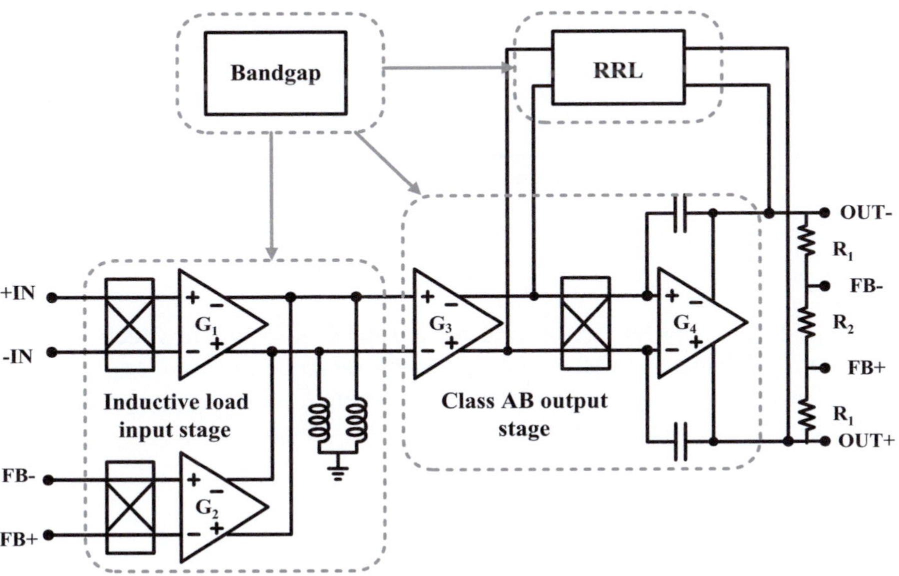

Fig. 3.16 Block diagram of a novel IA

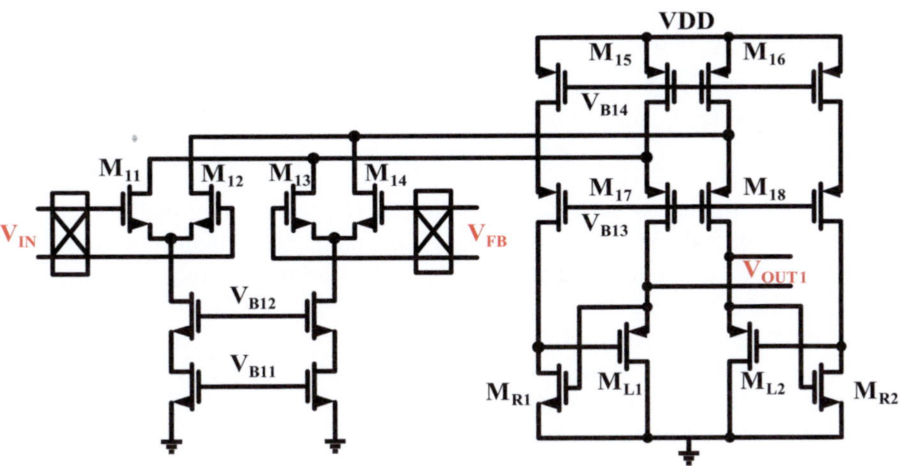

Fig. 3.17 The bandpass input stage circuit

The input stage of the IA is a bandpass amplifier that is realized using active inductors [12]. Its schematic is shown in Fig. 3.17. $M_{R1,2}$ is set in the linear region. It works as a resistor between the gate of transistor $M_{L1,2}$ and ground. Seen from the source of $M_{L1,2}$, an active inductance L is formed. The inductance and the output capacitance constitute bandpass load impedance, and a bandpass amplifier is thus realized.

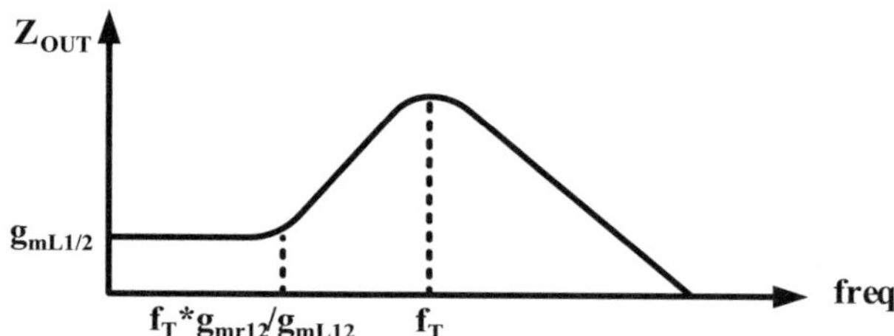

Fig. 3.18 Amplitude frequency response of Z_{OUT}

The inductance of the active inductor is shown in (3.14), in which f_T is the characteristic frequency of $M_{L1,2}$, and $g_{mR1,2}$ is the transconductance of $M_{R1/2}$, respectively. The expression of f_T is shown in (3.15), where $C_{GS1,2}$ and $g_{mL1,2}$ are the gate–source capacitance and the transconductance of $M_{L1,2}$, respectively.

$$L \approx \frac{1}{2\pi f_T g_{mR1,2}} \tag{3.14}$$

$$f_T \approx \frac{g_{mL1,2}}{2\pi C_{GS1,2}} \tag{3.15}$$

The output impedance is written in (3.16). Again, g_{mx} and r_{ox} are the transconductance and the output resistance of each transistor M_x. C_{OUT} is the total load capacitance at the output node.

$$Z_{OUT} \approx \left[\left(r_{o11,12} \;/\!/\; r_{o13,14} \;/\!/\; r_{o15,16} \right) g_{m17,18} r_{o17,18} \right] /\!/ \left(\frac{1}{g_{mL1,2}} + sL \right) /\!/ \frac{1}{sC_{OUT}} \tag{3.16}$$

At the low-frequency end, Z_{OUT} is as low as $1/g_{mL1,2}$. At the middle frequency range where the inductor takes effect, Z_{OUT} turns high. At the high frequency, Z_{OUT} drops again due to the load capacitance C_{OUT}. The amplitude frequency response of Z_{OUT} is drawn in Fig. 3.18.

The input transistors M_{11}–M_{14} work in the weak inversion region so as to acquire a high g_m/I_{DS} ratio. The quiescent current is carefully chosen to meet the noise requirement. Small transistor sizes can be chosen to increase input impedances while the 1/f noise and offsets can still be filtered by the bandpass stage, and this is one benefit of this structure.

The circuit of the second stage (actually the output stage) is shown in Fig. 3.19. It consists of a folded cascode input stage, a class-AB output stage, and a common mode feedback (CMFB) circuit. Its input is V_{OUT1} which is just the output of the first stage, and its output is V_{OUT2}. The second modulator is put at the drains of input transistors M_{21} and M_{22} and the two NMOS transistors M_{25} and M_{26}, which are used as current source. The offsets of transistors M_{21}–M_{26} are also modulated to the chopper frequency and they are separated from the signal in frequency domain.

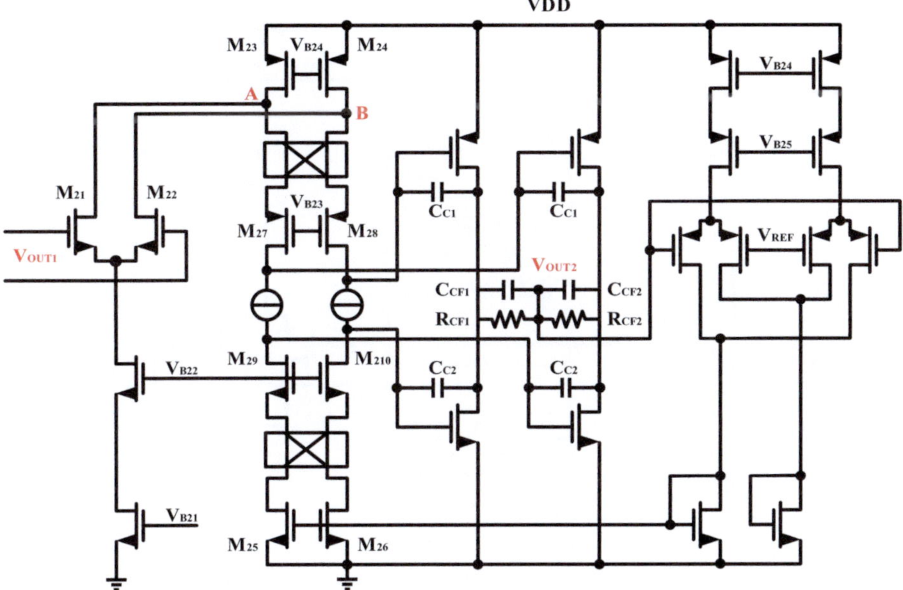

Fig. 3.19 IA output stage circuit

Moreover, the signal acquires more gain between the two modulators. So, the offsets and the low-frequency noises induced by transistors, which are behind the second modulator, have less influence on the signal when it is modulated back to low frequency.

As the offsets and 1/f noises of M_{21}–M_{26} have critical effects on output ripple, they are designed with large size without sacrificing performance. On the other hand, the 1/f noises of transistors M_{27}–M_{210} have influence on the corner frequency of input referred noise and the residual offset. They also have large W/L ratio.

A Class AB driver is used to save static power consumption and drive rail-to-rail output voltage. Traditional CMFB circuit, which has limited input voltage range, is not suitable to be used here. The output differential voltages are averaged by resistors R_{CF1} and R_{CF2} first. Then the common mode voltage with appropriate voltage range is processed in the following circuit. The capacitors C_{CF1} and C_{CF2}, which connect with resistors in parallel, improve the stability of the loop.

In the second stage, the offsets of transistors, which lay between the bandpass amplifier and the second modulator, i.e., M_{21}–M_{26}, will generate output ripple. They are not suppressed by the bandpass amplifier. So, an RRL circuit [24] is adopted to further reduce the ripple. Its block diagram is shown in Fig. 3.20.

The output signal V_{OUT2} is filtered by the AC couple capacitor C_{FB}. The high-frequency chopper ripple is extracted from the low-frequency signal. The ripple is chopped down to DC by modulators SW_{31}–SW_{34} and amplified by a gain boosting amplifier, which consists of M_{33}–M_{310}, two auxiliary amplifiers A_{31} and A_{32}, and large load capacitor C_{INT}. The amplifier has a quite low dominant pole and acts like an integrator. The low frequency ripple is integrated to a near constant voltage

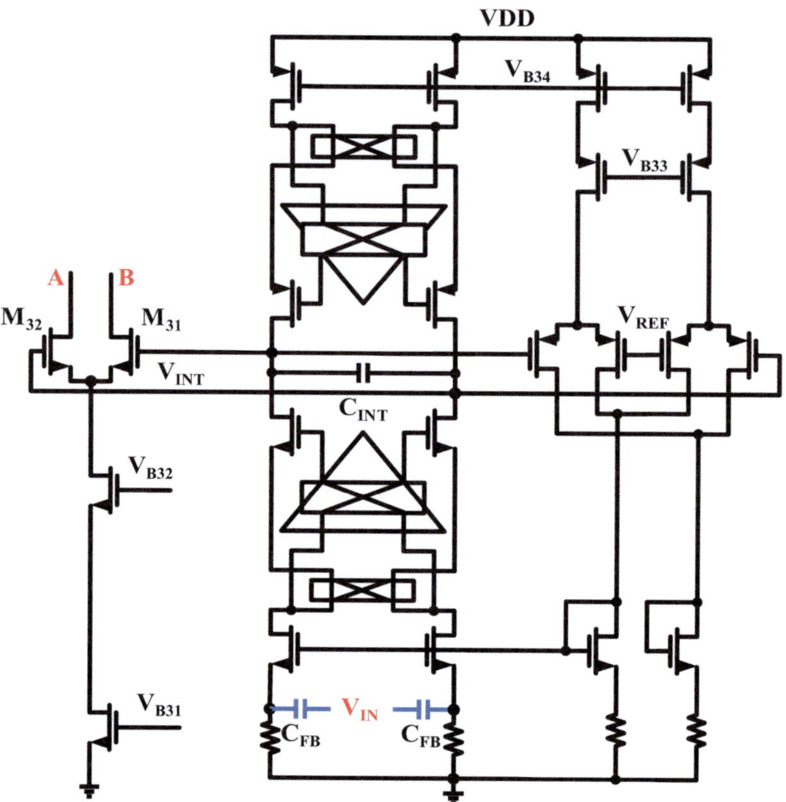

Fig. 3.20 Ripple reduction loop (RRL) circuit

VINT and then is transferred to current by M_{31} and M_{32} to cancel out the offset, which is mainly generated by transistors M_{21}–M_{26}. The right part is the CMFB circuit of the amplifier.

The RRL circuit does not limit drive capability. It has low power consumption and is easy to be realized on chip. By the bandpass amplifier and the RRL circuit, the offset and low-frequency noise that will generate output ripple are decreased tremendously.

Simulation and Verification

The presented IA has been designed in 0.18 μm CMOS technology with a 2.6 V power supply. It has a fixed closed loop gain of 40 dB and can be used to amplify a weak input voltage signal down to a few millivolts.

The output residual offset and the ripple caused by the equivalent input referred offsets (EIRO) at different nodes in the IA are simulated using the block diagram

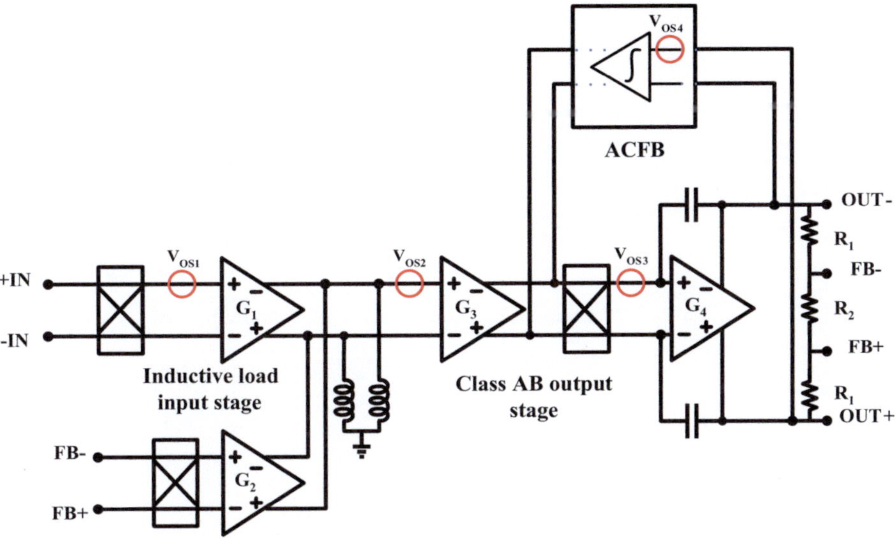

Fig. 3.21 The block diagram of the IA considering offsets at different nodes

Table 3.1 The residual offset and the ripple caused by offsets

Offset	Presetting voltage (mV)	Output residual offset (nV)	Output ripple (nV)
V_{OS1}	10	2.51	8.02
V_{OS2}	10	0.17	0.84
V_{OS3}	10	8304	19.70
V_{OS4}	10	1.37	63.64

shown in Fig. 3.21. V_{OS1} is the EIRO caused by the bandpass stage, V_{OS2} is the EIRO caused by the transistors of the output stage that lay before the second modulator, V_{OS3} is the EIRO caused by the rest of transistors of the second stage that are after the second modulator, and V_{OS4} is the EIRO caused by the amplifier in the RRL circuit.

The offset at different nodes have different contribution to the overall residual offset and the overall ripple. The simulation results are summarized in Table 3.1. Normally, the output ripple appears mainly due to V_{OS1}. By the bandpass amplifier, 10 mV V_{OS1} only leads to 8.02 nV output ripple. Meanwhile, the effects of V_{OS2} can also be neglected by using the RRL circuit. On the contrary, V_{OS3} and V_{OS4} are the main causes for the output ripple. That means the latter part G_4 of the output stage and the integrator in the RRL should be carefully designed with best matching. V_{OS3} is also the crucial factor for the residual offset. The usage of the bandpass amplifier increases the effective gain of the signal and thus the influence of V_{OS3} is reduced as well.

As shown in Fig. 3.22, the open-loop gain of the circuit is 150 dB and a peaking is found at 100 kHz, which is the chopper frequency. The peaking is caused by the

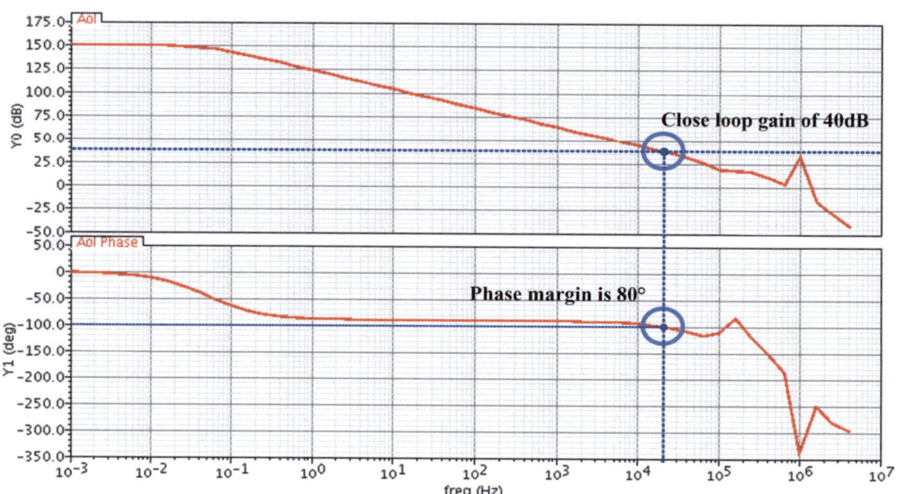

Fig. 3.22 Simulated open-loop gain of the IA

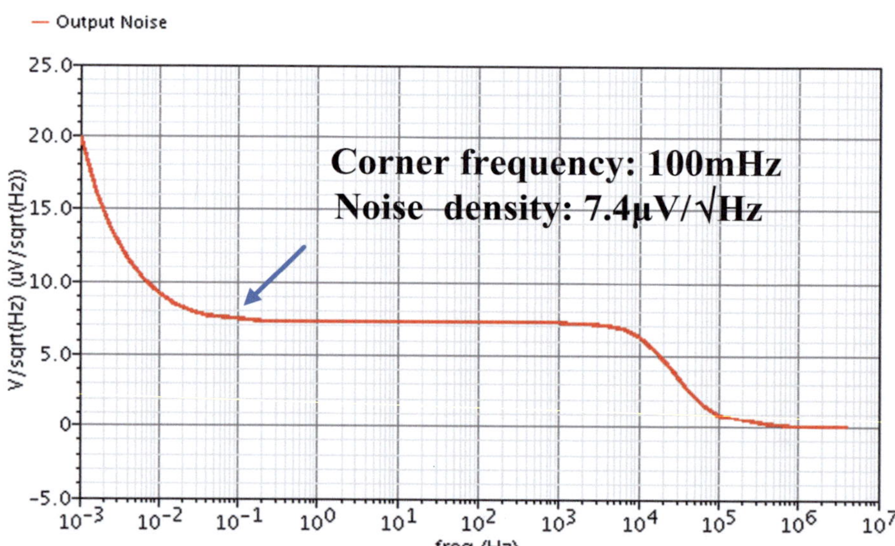

Fig. 3.23 simulated IA output referred noise spectrum

bandpass input stage. But the amplifier can still work stably at 40 dB with about 80°
phase margin. The noise spectrum is drawn in Fig. 3.23. The corner frequency
between 1/f noise and thermal noise is 0.1 Hz with an input referred noise density
of 74 nV/$\sqrt{\text{Hz}}$.

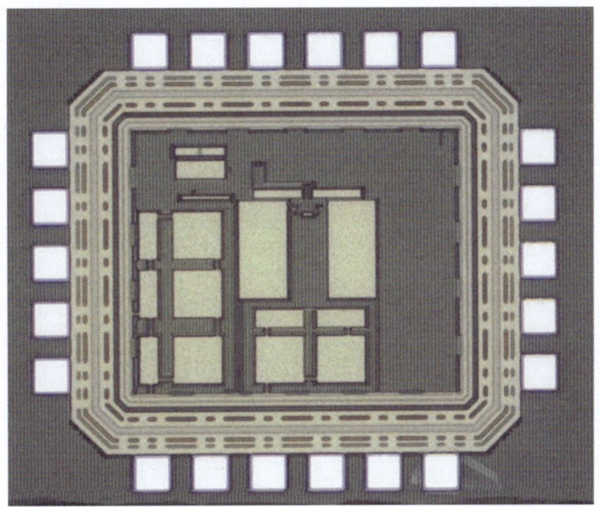

Fig. 3.24 Micrograph of the IA test chip

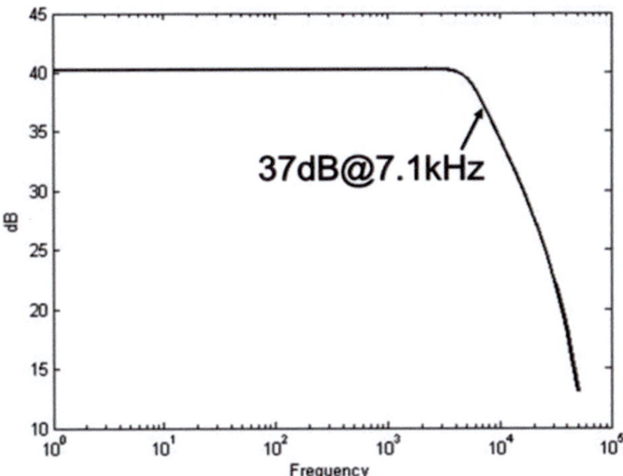

Fig. 3.25 Measured IA closed loop gain versus frequency

Measurement Results

The IA test chip was fabricated in 0.18 µm CMOS technology. The chip micrograph is shown in Fig. 3.24. The core area is only 0.16 mm^2.

The measured closed loop gain is shown in Fig. 3.25. The IA has a gain of 40 dB and its BW is 7.1 kHz.

The output referred noise spectrum is shown in Fig. 3.26. It is 7.4 µV/$\sqrt{\text{Hz}}$ at 0.1 Hz, which is in accordance with the simulation result. The first peaking in the figure is at 50 Hz, which is the power line interference. The second peaking is at

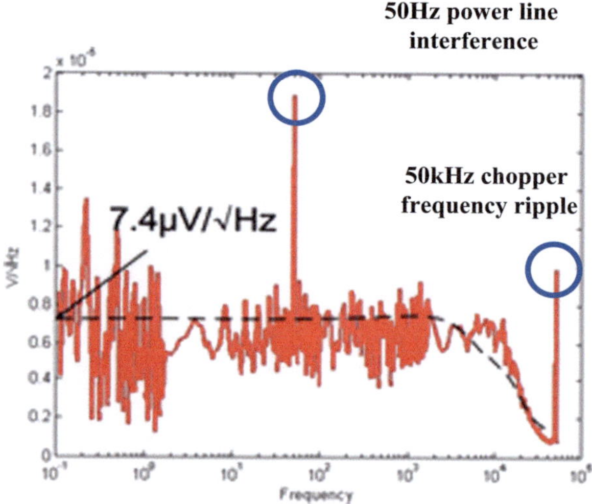

Fig. 3.26 Measured IA output noise

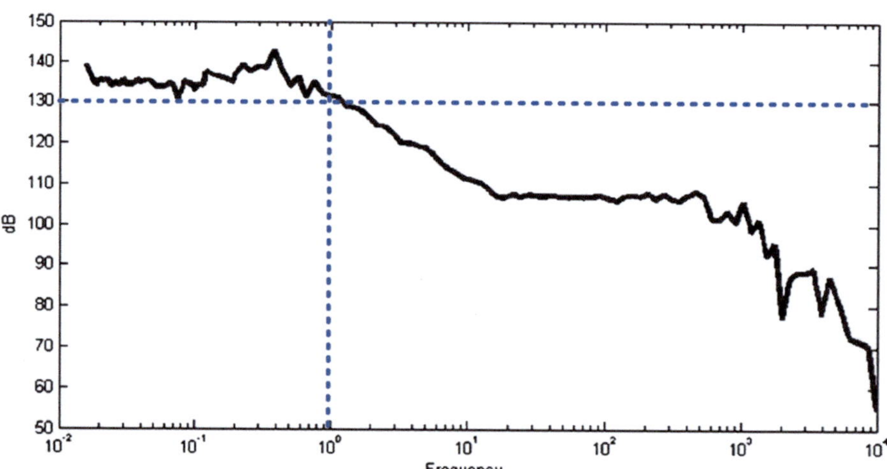

Fig. 3.27 Measured IA CMRR versus frequency

50 kHz, which is the chopper frequency. From Fig. 3.26, it can be seen that the ripple level is reduced to the noise floor.

The CMRR of the IA is shown in Fig. 3.27. The CMRR is higher than 130 dB below 1 Hz and the measured input referred residual offset is 3 µV. Noise efficiency factor (NEF) is usually used to measure the performance of the IA. The presented IA has an NEF of 15.5. The NEF is a bit high because the chip occupies small area by using small transistors and it has low power consumption, which means the thermal noise would be high. The performance of the IA is summarized in Table 3.2.

Table 3.2 IA measurement performance summary

Technology	0.18 μm CMOS
Active chip area	0.16 mm^2
Supply voltage	2.6 V
Quiescent current	30 μA
Gain (fixed)	40 dB
BW	7.1 kHz
Input referred noise @ 0.1 Hz	74 nV/$\sqrt{\text{Hz}}$
Input referred residual offset	3 μV
CMRR below 1 Hz	>130 dB
NEF	15.5

In summary, the chopper current feedback IA presented in this subsection has a bandpass amplification stage and RRL circuit, which could suppress the output voltage ripple and the residual offset. The IA is fabricated in 0.18 μm CMOS technology. The measurement results show that it has the advantages of small chip area, low power consumption, low ripple, low residual offset, and high CMRR. The IA is suitable to be used in low-power wireless medical and health care application systems.

3.3 Digitization Circuit

3.3.1 Design Considerations

For a digital biomedical sensor, a digitization circuit is required to convert the analog output of the sensor interface circuit, which is usually a voltage signal or a current signal, into a digital signal. When implementing a wireless medical/health care system, the most important performances for a sensor digitization circuit are resolution, sampling rate, and power consumption. Design trade-off has been made among these key parameters.

There are many choices to design a biomedical digitization circuit. Traditionally, an ADC can be used. Since most of the biomedical sensors have very limited signal bandwidth, the required ADC sampling rate is relatively low and is usually at the order of 10~10,000 sample/second (sps). Thus, the designers can choose not only low speed but also low-power ADC structures for biomedical sensors.

- For digitization resolution of ~12 bits, the Nyquist rate ADCs such as the successive-approximation (SAR) ADC or the cyclic ADC might be a good choice.
- For digitization resolution beyond 12 bits, the Σ-Δ ADC utilizing the oversampling and noise-shaping techniques is usually used.

It should be noted that the Σ–Δ ADC for high-resolution digitization has some intrinsic drawbacks associated with the Σ–Δ modulation and decimation filtering, which may result in extra power consumption and lower the sample-by-sample performance.

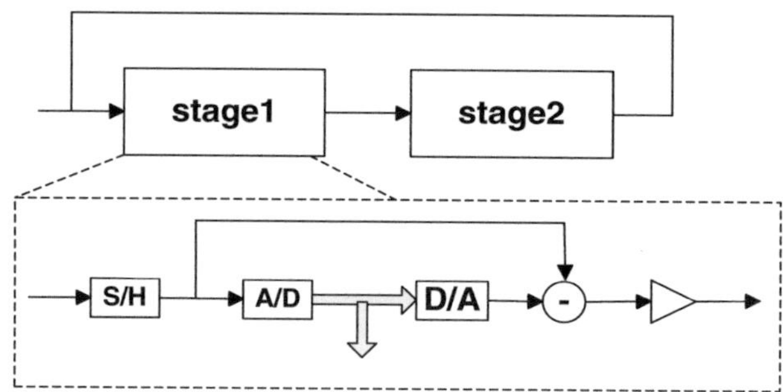

Fig. 3.28 Common architecture of cyclic ADC

For the low-speed biomedical sensor digitization requiring high resolution, there are some other digitization circuits, such as the analog-to-time converter (ATC) and the analog-to-frequency converter (AFC) that can be used to achieve both high resolution and low power consumption under low sampling rate. The voltage–pulse converter (VPC) digitizer that will be introduced in Sect. 3.3.3 is an example. In the VPC design, the method of multisteps quantization can be used to obtain a high resolution under a relative high update rate with low power consumption. Self-calibrating operation for offset cancellation helps to improve the conversion linearity.

The following part of this section will provide two digitizer design examples that can be used for biomedical sensors.

3.3.2 A Cyclic Analog-to-Digital Conversion Circuit

In this subsection, the circuit of an 8-bit 4 ksps cyclic ADC in a CMOS technology will be discussed. The cyclic ADS is also featured with small die area.

Cyclic ADC Architecture

The architecture of an 8-bit cyclic ADC is illustrated in Fig. 3.28. The 8-bit cyclic ADC is composed of two conversion stages, each stage can be a 1-bit conversion stage. For the conversion, each conversion cycle is divided into eight equal phases, and each phase will output 1-bit code. The input signal will be sampled by the first stage during the first phase of each conversion cycle. Then, the output of the second stage will be feedback as the input of the first stage at the third, fifth, and seventh phases for the cyclic operation. Thus, the 8-bit digital output code can be generated for each conversion cycle.

Each stage consists of a sample-and-hold (S/H) circuit, a single-bit analog-to-digital (A/D) converter and a digital-to-analog (D/A) converter, an analog subtractor, and an $x2$ amplifier [25].

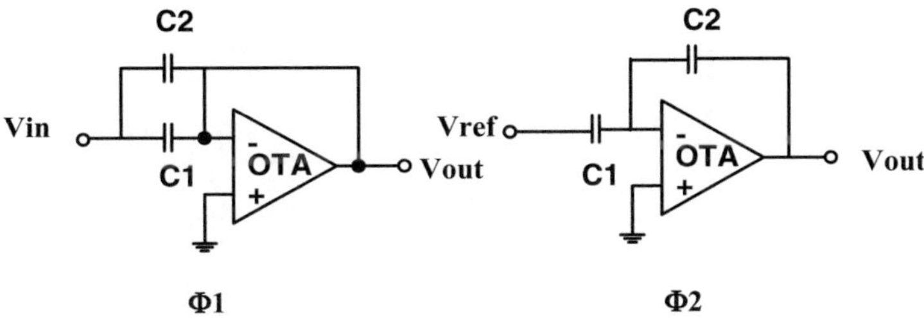

Fig. 3.29 MDAC architecture

The functions of the S/H, D/A, subtractor, and $x2$ amplifier can be combined together and performed using a multiplying DAC circuit (MDAC) as shown in Fig. 3.29. The commonly used switched-capacitor structure can be adopted here. The function of one-bit A/D can be accomplished by the comparator. In the MDAC, all the operation is achieved via charge transfer using a common capacitor array.

The operation of an MDAC within one operation cycle can also be divided into two phases, namely, Φ_1 and Φ_2. In the sampling phase Φ_1, the input signal charges the top plate of the capacitors C_1 and C_2, and the charge on C_1 and C_2 can be expressed as:

$$Q_{\phi 1} = -V_{in} \cdot (C_1 + C_2)$$
(3.17)

In phase Φ_2 for subtraction and amplification, the charge will be redistributed on the top plate of C_1 and C_2. Assuming the bottom plate of C_1 is connected to V_{ref}, the charge on C_1 and C_2 can be expressed as:

$$Q_{\phi 2} = -V_{ref} \cdot C_1 + V_{out} \cdot C_2$$
(3.18)

in which V_{out} is the output voltage at the end of phase Φ_2.

By equating (3.17) and (3.18), the output voltage V_{out} can be obtained as:

$$V_{out} = \frac{C_1 + C_2}{C_2} V_{in} - \frac{C_1}{C_2} V_{ref}$$
(3.19)

If $C_1 = C_2$, the output voltage can be expressed as:

$$V_{out} = 2V_{in} - V_{ref}$$
(3.20)

Thus, the functions of the S/H, DAC, subtraction, and $x2$ amplifier are accomplished just by the MDAC.

1.5-bit Stage

In Fig. 3.28, each conversion stage is a 1-bit converter. Actually, the conversion stage can be a multibit converter, such as a 1.5-bit converter [26]. The 1.5-bit stage has shown many advantages in the design of the pipeline ADC.

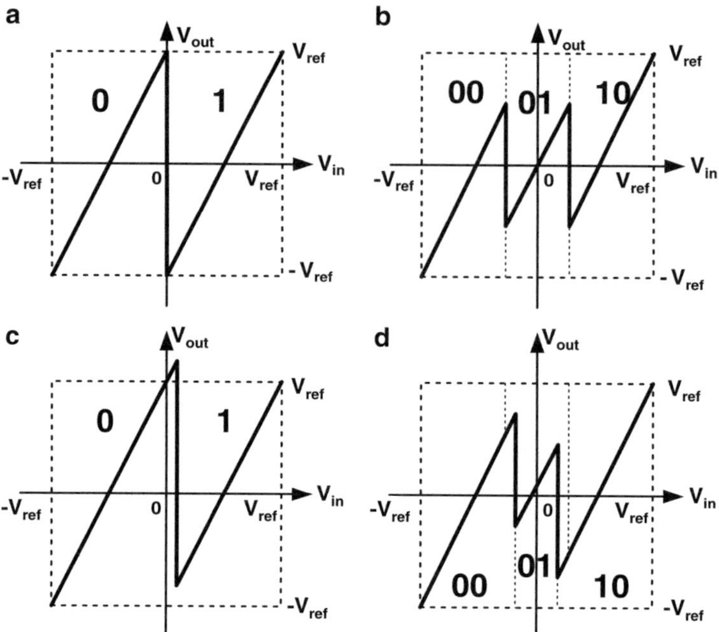

Fig. 3.30 MDAC transfer curves of 1-bit stage (**a**, **c**) vs. 1.5-bit stage (**b**, **d**)

It also has remarkable performance in the cyclic ADC. The 1.5-bit stage is a modification of the 1-bit stage. Some redundancy is built in the 1.5-bit stage to provide a large tolerance to mismatching and offsets. Especially, the demand on the comparator offset voltage is alleviated greatly in the 1.5-bit stage. Figure 3.30a, b illustrates the ideal transfer curve of the MDAC with 1-bit and 1.5-bit stage, respectively. With the comparator offset present, the output of the 1-bit stage can easily fall beyond the effective voltage range as shown in Fig. 3.30c, and some unrecoverable error is generated. On the contrary, in the 1.5-bit stage, the error caused by the comparator offset voltage will not result in any over range problem as shown in Fig. 3.30d. The MDAC output in the 1.5-bit stage will not exceed the correct range $-V_{ref} \sim +V_{ref}$ when the offset of the comparator is between $-0.25\ V_{ref}$ and $+0.25\ V_{ref}$. With the help of digital correction algorithm which eliminates the redundancy later, the final digitization result can be calculated. It can also be further proven that the comparator offset voltage in the proceeding stages will not have any effect on the ADC transition points. This 1.5-bit architecture greatly simplifies the design of comparator. A low-power, high-speed, but high-offset dynamic comparator can be used in an MDAC.

Differential Implementation

The fully differential circuit could reject the common-mode disturbances generated by the digital circuits, clock drivers, etc. A single-ended to differential-ended transfer circuit is needed because the input signal from the sensor interface circuit is usually single ended.

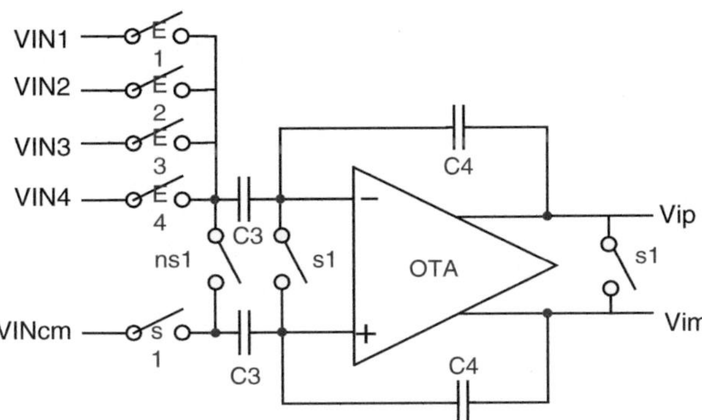

Fig. 3.31 Single-ended to differential-ended transform circuit

The switched-capacitor architecture is used here again as shown in Fig. 3.31. Figure 3.31 actually shows a single-ended to differential circuit with four input channels. The switch control signals $E_1\sim E_4$ decide which channel will be selected and sampled at a certain time. The output of the transfer can be expressed as:

$$V_{ip} - V_{im} = \frac{C_4}{C_3}\left(V_{IN} - V_{INcm}\right) \tag{3.21}$$

The major part of the fully differential cyclic ADC circuit including the two main stages, the comparator and the digital redundancy correction circuits, are shown in Fig. 3.32. For each conversion cycle, at the first 1/8 phase, the single-ended input will be converted into differential-ended using the circuit in Fig. 3.31. Then the differential signals will be sent to the input of the first stage at the second 1/8 phase for conversion. Other modules such as the reference voltage generation circuit are omitted here. The corresponding switch controlling sequences are shown in Fig. 3.33.

The power consumption of ADC consists of two parts, the analog power and the digital power. The analog power is mainly consumed by the operational amplifiers, which are set by the biasing current. They are used to settle the analog output to the desired accuracy. The digital power is in proportion to the frequency of the input clock. The power consumption can be greatly reduced by two means. First, the current of the analog part can be turned off by closing the bias. Almost no power will be consumed by the analog circuit in this condition. Second, the clock-gating method can be used to close the clock signal of the digital part. There is no activity associated with reloading of registers in the digital part, thus no power. Only leakage current will lead to some tiny power consumption in sleep mode.

Circuit Design

For the cyclic ADC architecture presented above, it can be seen that the operational amplifiers and the comparator are the two key modules of the ADC. The detailed circuit of these two blocks will be discussed as follows.

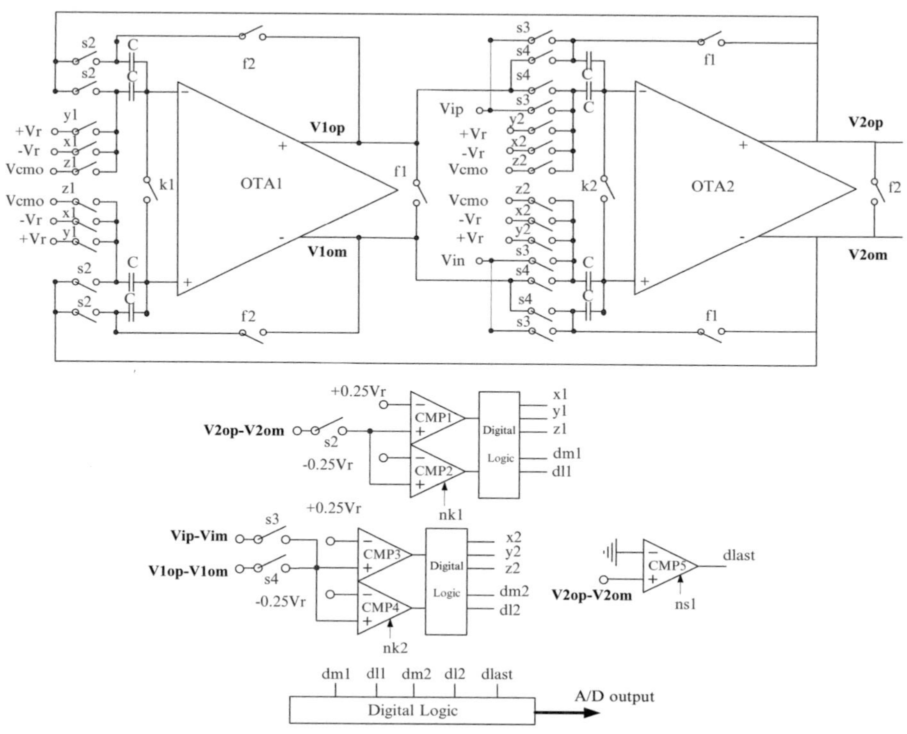

Fig. 3.32 Fully differential cyclic ADC circuit

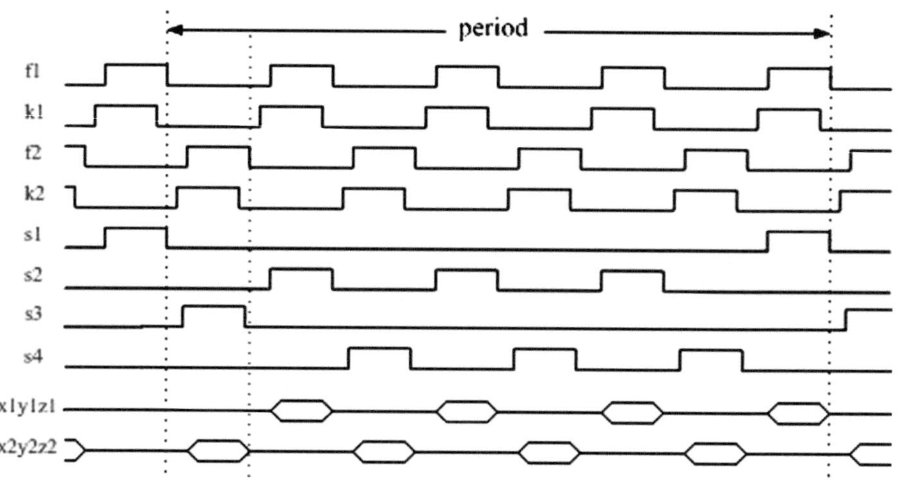

Fig. 3.33 Fully differential cyclic ADC circuit switch control sequences

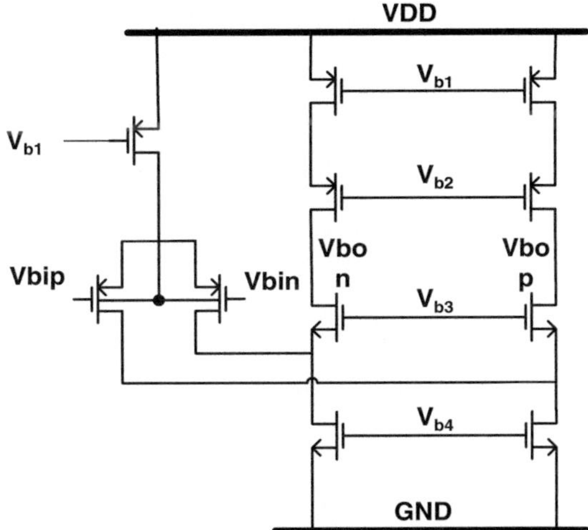

Fig. 3.34 Folded-cascode fully differential operational amplifier (OTA)

The operational amplifiers are used in the MDAC, the single-ended to differential-ended converter and the reference voltage generator. The operational amplifier designed here is based on the fully differential folded-cascode structure as shown in Fig. 3.34. This structure has good compromise between low power consumption and large output swing. A high-swing biasing circuit provides the four biasing voltages for the operational amplifiers. A switched-capacitors common-mode feedback circuit is also integrated to stabilize the common output voltage and reduce clock feed through distortion.

In a normal working mode, most of the power is consumed by the operational amplifiers. Small W/L ratios of all MOS transistors are selected in order to get a relatively high transconductance g_m under the condition of low current. Large L also helps to reduce the input offset voltage. Low overdriven voltage of the input transistors is a good choice for a high DC gain with low power. The decrease in the bandwidth resulted from the low $V_{gs} - V_{th}$ is not critical here, as the circuit works in quite low speed and the operational amplifier bandwidth requirement is also low.

The layout of the operational amplifier should be optimized carefully. The input transistors and current mirror are placed in a common centroid style to lower the mismatch. In this way, the effects of global layout gradients can be averaged out. The dummy transistors can be added to eliminate the mismatch of the peripheral devices.

The postlayout simulation shows that the designed operational amplifier has a DC gain of 70 dB, a band-width of 140 kHz under the worst case situation. The phase margin exceeds 70°. Each amplifier with biasing circuit consumes power less than 1 µW.

The dynamic comparator utilizing the latch structure used in the MDAC is shown in Fig. 3.35. This structure has the advantage of low power and high speed. The input offset voltage is not a critical restrict of the ADC due to the adoption of 1.5-bit stage.

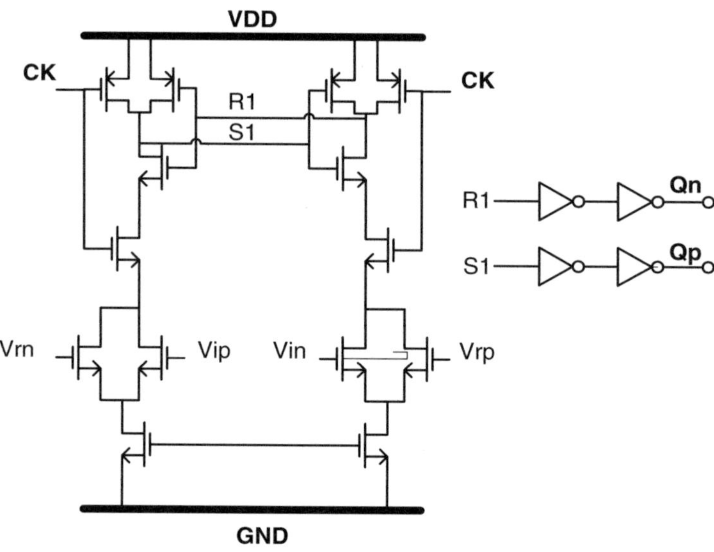

Fig. 3.35 Dynamic comparator

Measurement Results

The cyclic ADC was fabricated in a 0.18 μm 1P6M CMOS technology. Figure 3.36 shows the micrograph of the test chip. The core of the ADC including both the analog and digital parts occupies only 0.12 mm². In the measurements, the supply voltages AVDD and DVDD were both set to 1.8 V.

The code density test was conducted using a full-swing sinusoidal input with amplitude of 1.8 V. A sample frequency of 4 kHz is implemented, which satisfies the demand of many wireless medical/health care systems. More than one million samples were taken. The measured integral nonlinearity (INL) and differential non-linearity (DNL) of the ADC are shown in Figs. 3.37 and 3.38, respectively. The INL and DNL is in the range of −0.3/0.2 LSB and −0.25/0.27 LSB, respectively.

Figure 3.39 plots the measured output spectrum of the ADC under the sample frequency of 4 kHz. The amplitude and frequency of the input sine signal were set to −0.15 dbFS, 304.7 Hz. The result shows that the ADC has an SFDR of 57.8 dB and an SNDR of 47.1 dB. It corresponds to an effective number of bit (ENOB) of 7.53 bit under this sample frequency, using (3.22).

$$ENOB = \frac{SNDR\left(dB\right)-1.76}{6.02} \tag{3.22}$$

In the normal working mode, the total power dissipation of the cyclic ADC is 12.5 μW with 1.8 V power supply and a 4-kHz sampling frequency. When the ADC is in the sleep mode, the total current drained from AVDD and DVDD is only 78 nA. It means that the ADC consumes less than 150 nW in the sleep mode.

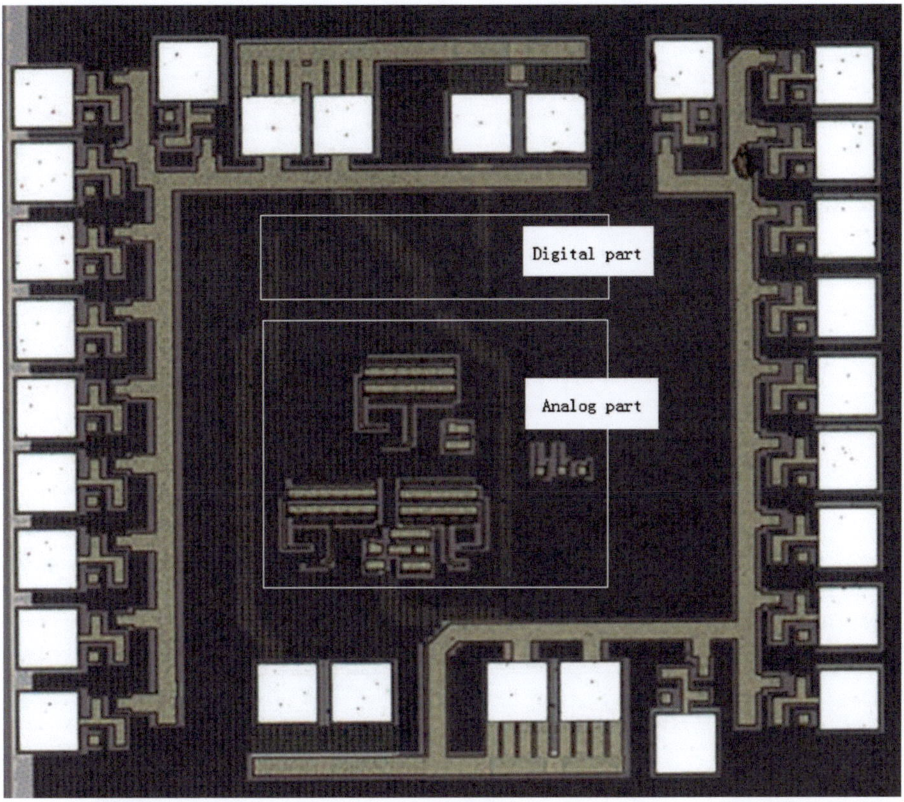

Fig. 3.36 Micrograph of the cyclic ADC test chip

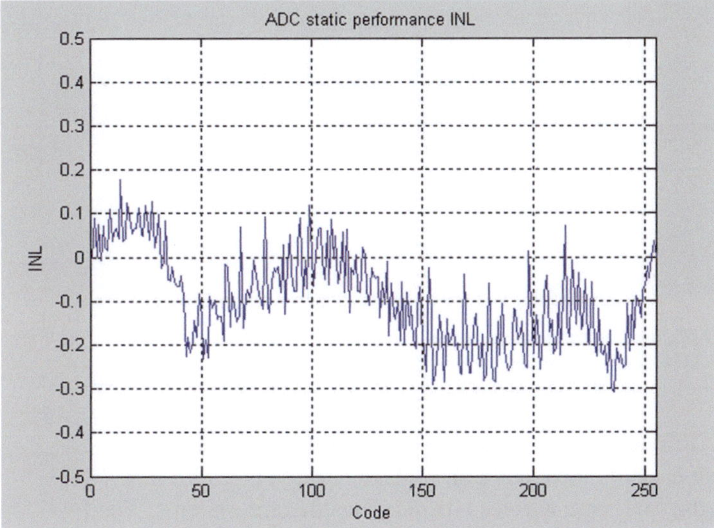

Fig. 3.37 Measured INL of the cyclic ADC

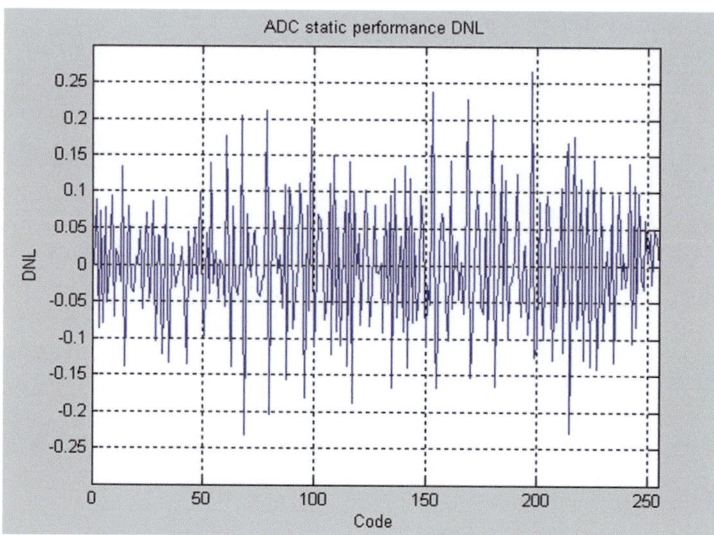

Fig. 3.38 Measured DNL of the cyclic ADC

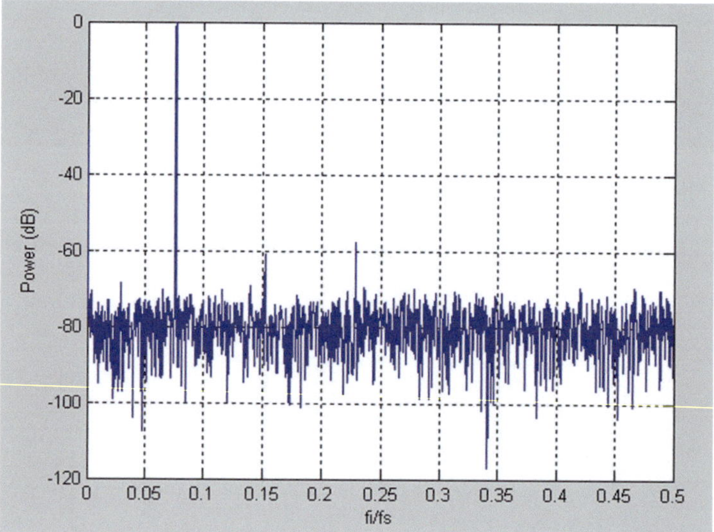

Fig. 3.39 Measured output spectrum of the cyclic ADC with the −0.15 dbFS, 304.7 Hz sinusoidal input and 4 kHz sample frequency

The ADC performance summary is given in Table 3.3.

In summary, this subsection presents the design of a 12.5 μW, 4 ksps, 8-bit cyclic ADC for the real-time wireless medical/health care systems. The two-stage cyclic architecture is adopted in the design. It has the characteristic of good balance

Table 3.3 Cyclic ADC performance summary

Supply voltage	1.8 V
Sample frequency	4 kHz
Input range	0~1.8 V
Power dissipation (norm working mode)	12.5 μW
Power dissipation (sleep mode)	0.15 μW
SFNR @ fin=304.7 Hz	57.8 dB
SNDR @ fin=304.7 Hz	47.1 dB
ENOB @ fin=304.7 Hz	7.53 bit
Max sample frequency	40 kHz, ENOB>7 bit
INL	0.3 LSB
DNL	0.27 LSB
Chip size (ADC core)	400 μm × 300 μm

between low power and small die area. Each stage consists of a sample-and-hold circuit, a single-bit AD convertor, a single-bit DA convertor, an analog subtractor, and an $x2$ amplifier. The S/H, DAC, subtraction, and $x2$ amplifier are combined in an MDAC. The 1.5-bit stage is utilized to simplify the design of comparator. The operational amplifier and dynamic comparator are designed with careful optimization. Experimental results show that the ADC chip under 0.18 μm 1P6M CMOS process consumes only 12.5 μW with a sampling rate of 4 ksps and 7.53-bit ENOB in the working mode. By turning off the biasing of the analog part and clock-gating the digital part, the ADC consumes less than 150 nW in the sleep mode. The low power and small size make it possible to further integrate the ADC inside a wireless medical/health care SOC.

3.3.3   Voltage–Pulse Conversion

A voltage–pulse converter (VPC) digitizer transforms the sensor interface output signal into the pulse signal. The presented VPC in this subsection has a wide input dynamic range (up to 350 pF for capacitive sensors). Its update rate is not quite high (around 1,000 sample per second with one single channel), but this is acceptable for wireless medical/health care applications as the sensor data rate is relatively low in these applications. The high-resolution VPC is achieved by using a multisteps quantization method. It is a blend of counting quantization and cyclic techniques in some extent.

Basic Operation

The basic operation of the VPC is illustrated in Fig. 3.40a, which consists of a sample-and-hold circuit, a 4-bit quantizer and a $\times 2^4$ amplifier.

First, the initial input signal $x_0[0]$ is sampled and subtracted by a constant value of $\Delta = FSR/2^4$ in each clock cycle, where FSR is full-scale range. As shown in Fig. 3.40b,

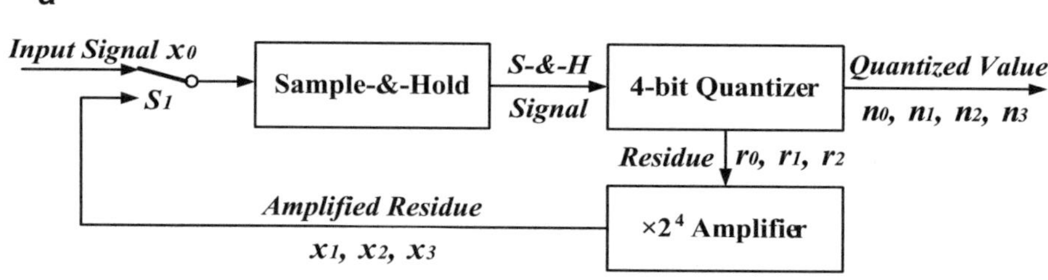

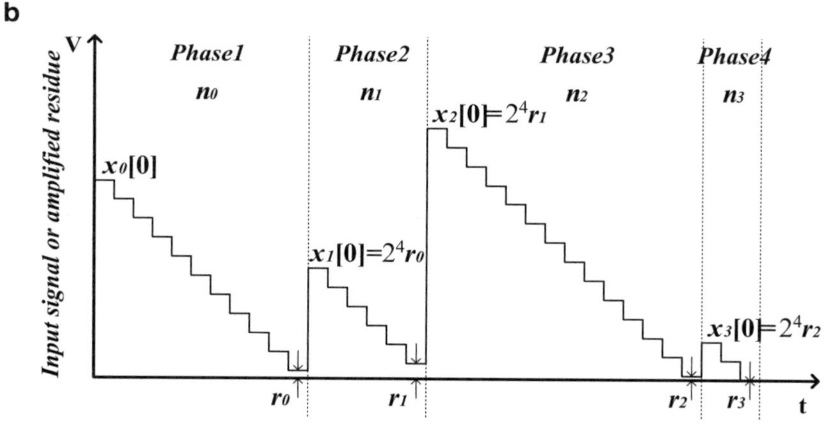

Fig. 3.40 Basic algorithm of voltage–pulse converter (VPC): (**a**) basic structure of VPC, (**b**) basic operation of VPC

this ramp-down counting operation stops when $x_0[n] - \Delta < 0$, where $n(0 \leq n \leq 15)$ is the number of clock cycles. The initial input signal $x_0[0]$ is converted into a 4-bit quantized value n_0, which is the number of clock cycles during the first quantization operation and corresponds to the most 4 significant bits of 16. At the end of the first counting phase, the residue $r_0 = x_0[n_0]$ is amplified by 2^4. Then the amplified residue $x_1[0] = 2^4 r_0$ is sampled and sent back to the 4-bit quantizer for the second conversion. By repeating this operation for four times, 4-bit quantized values n_0, n_0, n_0, and n_3, from the most to the least significant bits (LSB), are produced. The analog signal to be converted in next counting phase can be expressed as:

$$x_{m+1}[0] = 2^4 r_m = 2^4 x_m[n_m] = 2^4 \left(x_m[0] - n_m \Delta \right) \tag{3.23}$$

where $m = 0$, 1, or 2. The transfer function can be expressed as:

$$x_0 = \left(2^{12} n_0 + 2^8 n_1 + 2^4 n_2 + 2^0 n_3 \right) / 2^{12} \cdot \Delta \tag{3.24}$$

4×2^4 clock cycles is only required when all the input voltages at the beginning of all four conversion phases (i.e., $x_0[0]$, $x_1[0]$, $x_2[0]$ and $x_3[0]$) are equal to the

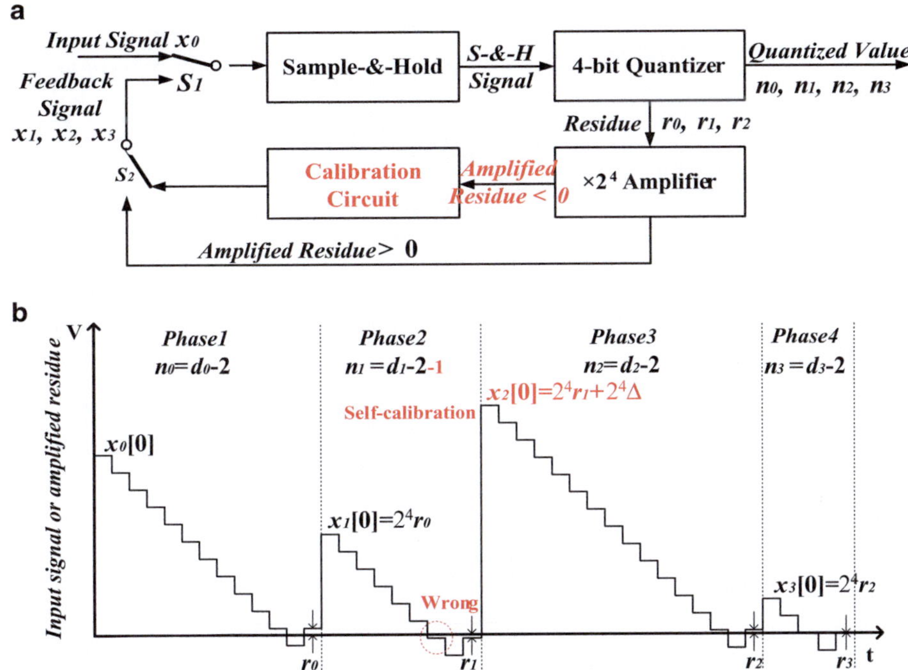

Fig. 3.41 Optimized algorithm of voltage–pulse converter (VPC): (**a**) optimized structure of VPC, (**b**) optimized operation of VPC

full-scale voltage. If the residues are correctly amplified (i.e., charge injection, and other errors are small), this multisteps quantization method can be quite powerful in increasing the resolution and reducing the conversion time.

Optimized Operation

Considering the implementation of circuitry, the VPC structure may be optimized as Fig. 3.41a, b. In a practical circuit, the state conversion is detected when $x_m[d]$ is smaller than 0, and the ramp-down operation stops. Then in the next clock cycle, Δ is added to $x_m[d]$, and the counting operation stops. The analog signal to be converted in next counting phase also can be expressed as (3.8), but n_m should be $d_m - 2$.

Additionally, due to the comparator's input offset or output hysteresis, a wrong rollover may occur when the converted analog signal is a little smaller than 0. In the second phase of Fig. 3.41b, $x_1[n_2+1]$ is wrongly judged to be larger than 0. As a result, the ramp-down operation stops at $x_1[n_2+3]$ instead of $x_1[n_2+2]$, which leads to a wrong quantization result n_1 and a wrong residue value r_1. Then r_1 is amplified by 2^4 times amplifier and a negative amplified residue is produced. This will cause VPC to fail in convergence, which is not allowed for further conversion. Thus, if $2^4 r_m$

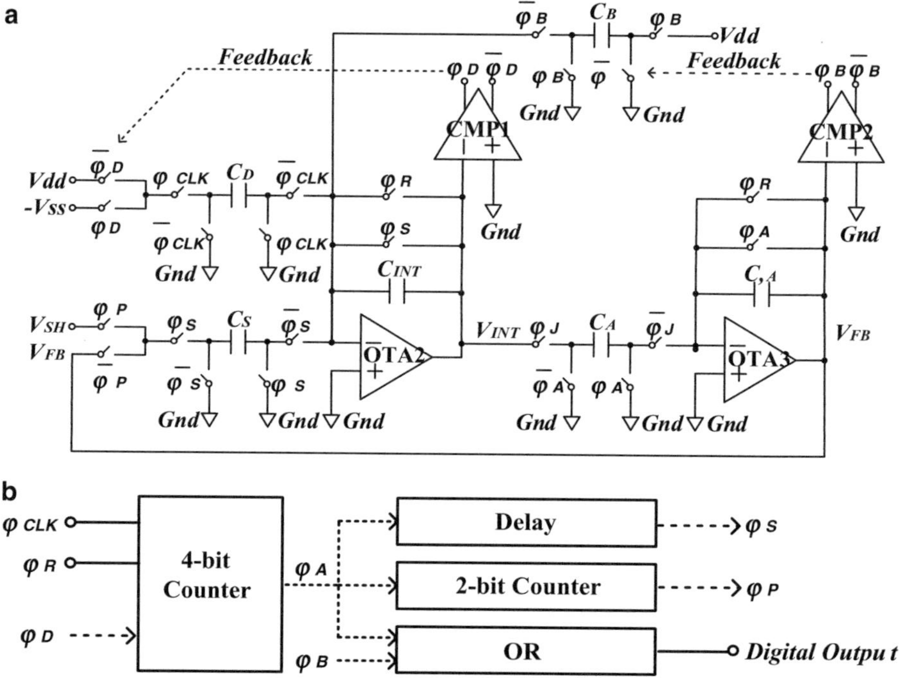

Fig. 3.42 Implementation of voltage–pulse converter (VPC): (a) detailed schematic of analog block, (b) basic schematic of timing control logic block

is smaller than 0, the analog signal to be converted in the next phase will automatically be calibrated to:

$$x_{m+1}[0] = 2^4 r_m + 2^4 \Delta \tag{3.25}$$

as shown in Fig. 3.41b. When it occurs, the quantized value of previous phase nm should be corrected with minus one clock cycles. This self-calibrating operation cancels the comparator's offset or hysteresis and improves the conversion linearity of VPC.

Circuitry Implementation

The detailed schematic of the presented voltage–pulse converter is shown in Fig. 3.42, which corresponds to the block diagram in Fig. 3.41a.

The 4-bit quantizer consists of operational transconductance amplifier OTA2, dynamic comparator CMP1, switched-capacitor C_S and C_D, and integration capacitor C_{INT}. The sample-and-hold operation is also completed by OTA2, C_S, and C_{INT}. $\times 2^4$ amplifier is realized by OTA3, switched-capacitor C_A, and feedback C_A'. The calibration circuit consists of CMP2 and switched-capacitor C_B. The timing control logic block is based on a 4-bit finite state machine, which is controlled by the output of CMP1 ϕ_D, the output of CMP2 ϕ_B, and the pulse of reset ϕ_R as described in Fig. 3.42b. The presented circuit works with dual supply ($V_{DD}/Gnd/V_{SS}$, i.e., V_{DD} = 0.9 V, Gnd = 0 V, V_{SS} = −0.9 V). The reference level of OTA and CMP is set to Gnd, which is equal to $(V_{DD}+V_{SS})/2$.

The voltage–pulses conversion starts with the pulse of reset ϕ_R. V_{SH} is sampled by C_S and held by $C_{INT} = C_S$. Then C_{INT} is discharged by $C_D = C_{INT}/18$ and V_{INT} ramps down with the step of $\Delta V = V_{DD}C_D/C_{INT}$. V_{INT} is expressed as:

$$V_{INT}\left[d\right] = V_{INT}\left[d-1\right] - d \cdot \Delta V \tag{3.26}$$

where d is the number of clock cycles for discharging, $V_{INT}[d]$ is the OPA2's output, and the initial value is $V_{INT}[1] = V_{SH} - \Delta V$. When $V_{INT}[d] < 0$, trip of V_{INT} beyond Gnd, CMP1 changes the state of ϕ_D. Then ΔV will be injected into C_{INT} by switched-capacitor C_D at next clock cycle. The first quantization phase will also be terminated at that clock cycle. With this ramp-down counting operation, V_{SH} is converted into a 4-bit quantized value of $n = d - 2(0 \leq n \leq 15)$, which corresponds to the most 4 significant bits of 16.

After the first quantization, the residue of the first 4-bit quantization $V_{INT0}[d]$ is amplified by $C_A/C_A' = 16$ under the control of ϕ_A to obtain a feedback voltage V_{FB}. A new converted signal $V_{INT1}[0] = V_{FB} - \Delta V$ is produced by ϕ_S. Then C_{INT} is discharged again and this 4-bit quantization procedure is repeated for another three times as is in Figs. 3.41b and 3.43. As a result, the intervals between two adjacent conversion phases represent four 4-bit quantized values in one complete conversion cycle. Compared to the previously reported Σ–Δ modulation-based or oscillator-based digitizers, the presented digitizer increases the resolution and reduces the conversion time with lower power consumption by introducing multisteps quantization method. Additionally, the OTAs, comparators, and capacitors of VPC are reused in every conversion operation. It greatly reduces the power and area consumption.

A simple low-power latched comparator structure is utilized in the comparator design [27] as shown in Fig. 3.44. The typical input offset of this type comparator is around 10–20 mV. Although the resolution requirement of main comparator CMP1 is only 4 bits, due to the comparator CMP1's input offset or output hysteresis, a wrong rollover may occur when $V_{INTm}[d] = V_{INTm}[d-1] + \Delta V$ is a little lower than Gnd. As a result, V_{FB} and $V_{INTm+1}[1]$ might be both lower than Gnd, which is not allowed for further conversion as shown in Figs. 3.41b and 3.43. The traditional principle for offset cancellation is to use a preamplifier to build up the input change to a sufficiently large value and then apply it to the latch. In this design, another comparator CMP2 is used to monitor the value of V_{FB}, which is 16 times of $V_{INTm+1}[d]$. At this situation, the 2^4 times amplifier is reused as an error amplifier. It amplifies the input value $V_{INTm}[d]$ to a sufficiently large value. If V_{FB} is lower than Gnd, the state of the pulse of borrow ϕ_B changes. A constant amount of charge $V_{DD}C_B$ will be injected into C_{INT} by switched-capacitor (SC) network C_B for self-calibration. $V_{INTm+1}[0]$ is adjusted as:

$$V_{INTm+1}\left[0\right] = V_{FB} - \Delta V + V_{DD}C_B / C_{INT} \tag{3.27}$$

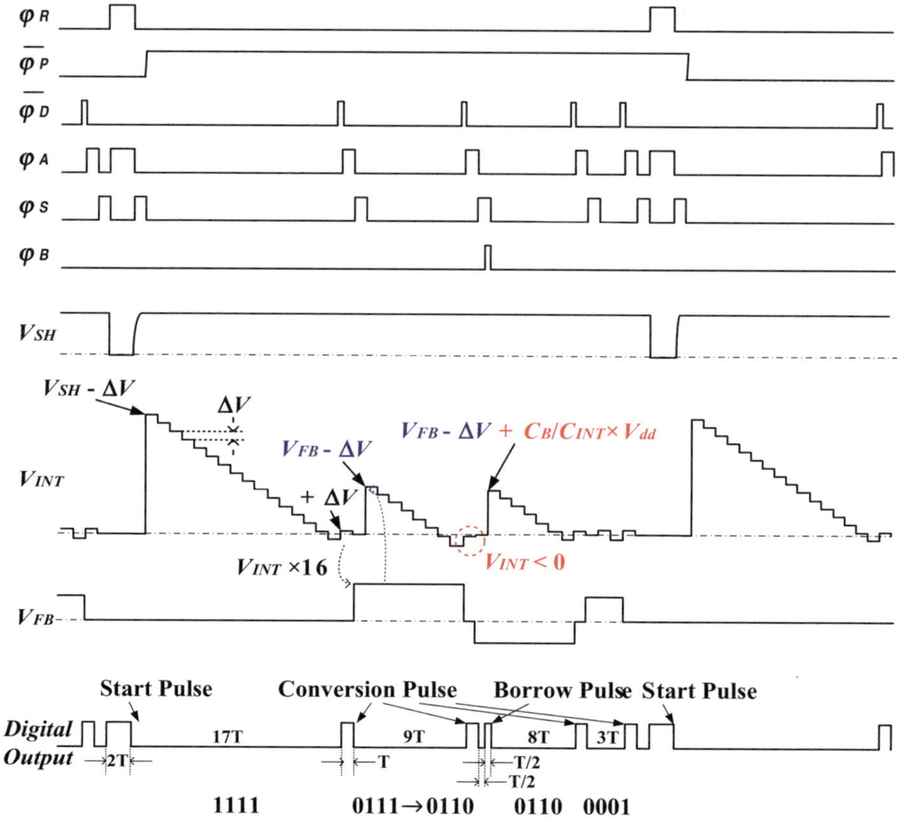

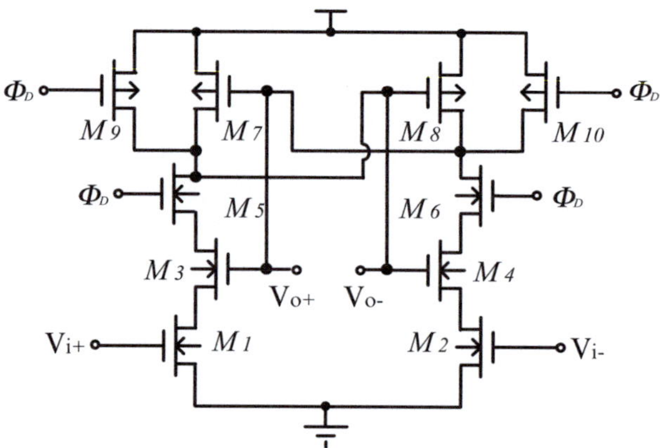

Fig. 3.43 Conversion operation of voltage–pulse converter

Fig. 3.44 The schematic of latched comparator CMP1 and CMP2

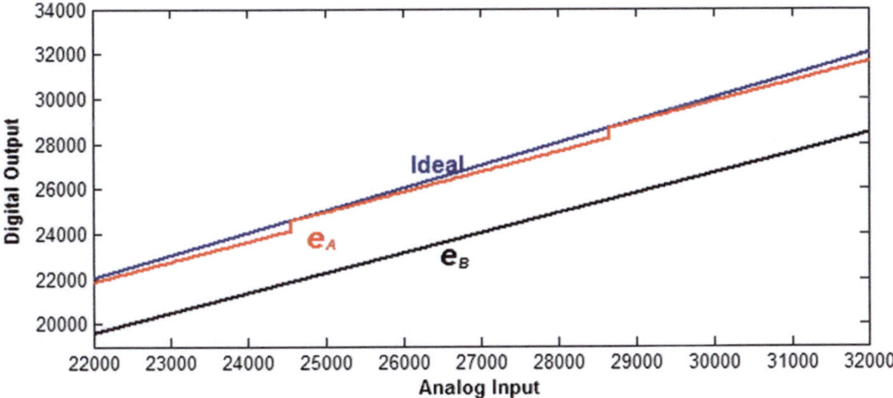

Fig. 3.45 Transfer curves of VPC with typical errors

where $C_B=16C_D$. $V_{INTm+1}[0]$ can continue the ramp-down counting operation after this correction. If CMP2 is not used, a negative V_{FB} will be sampled by C_S and then injected to C_{INT}. As a result, all the quantization value of remaining phases will be wrong ($d_m=2$). This self-calibrating operation cancels the comparator's offset or hysteresis and improves the conversion linearity.

Because the switched-capacitor structure has been used and the reference is fixed to *Gnd*, the accuracy and the resolution of the voltage–pulse converter only depend on the matching of the capacitors. These features ensure the circuit's robustness and the power-supply rejection performance.

Errors Analysis and Estimation

From (3.8) and (3.10), the performance of VPC is mainly limited by the gain 2^4 and the quantization step Δ. Thus, introduce two main parameters are introduced for the error analysis (1) the amplification error e_A and (2) the quantization step error e_B. The transfer function (3.24) upgrades to:

$$x_0 = \left[\left(2^4+e_A\right)^0 n_0 +\left(2^4+e_A\right)^{-1} n_1 +\left(2^4+e_A\right)^{-2} n_2 +\left(2^4+e_A\right)^{-3} n_3\right]$$
$$\cdot\left[\Delta/\left(1+e_B\right)\right] \tag{3.28}$$

The amplification error e_A is contributed by the mismatch of the circuit components as well as the finite gain and nonlinearity of the amplifiers. The quantization step error e_B is mainly due to the capacitor mismatches and charge injection.

From (3.28), the amplification error e_A and the quantization step error e_B both affect the transfer curve obviously as shown in Fig. 3.45. With the increase in the amplitude of analog input, the transfer curve deviates from the ideal curve periodically

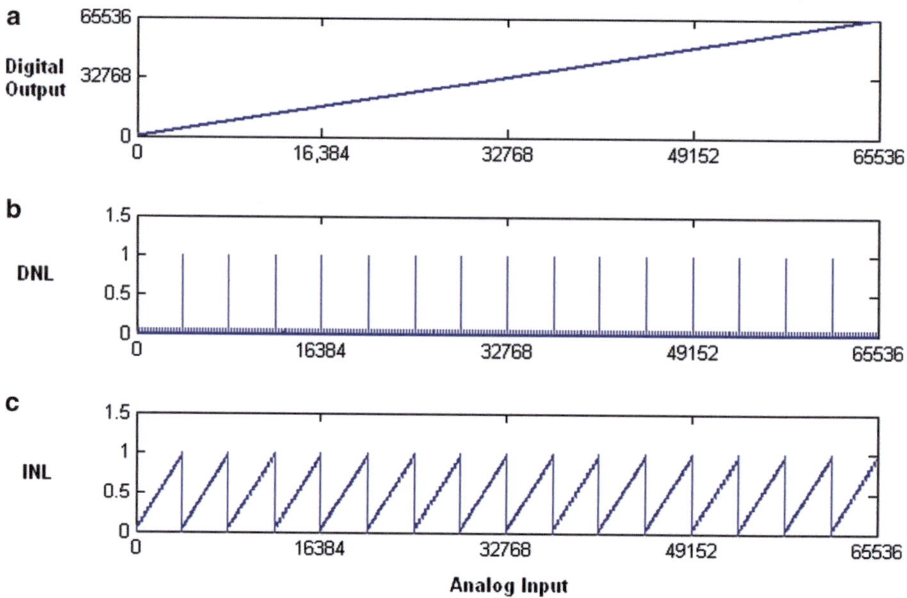

Fig. 3.46 The influence of amplification error e_A on DNL/INL: (**a**) transfer curve, (**b**) DNL, (**c**) INL. $e_A = 1/2^a$, where a is the accuracy of amplification. In these three figures, the accuracy is 12.1-bit

by the influence of e_A. e_B changes the slope of the transfer curves but does not affect the linearity. Therefore, e_A and e_B are utilized to estimate the nonlinearity and dynamic range, respectively.

The nonlinearity characteristic of the presented VPC structure is also simulated, only considering e_A, which is illustrated in Fig. 3.46.

The DNL is expressed as:

$$DNL = \left|\left(V_{D+1} - V_D\right) / V_{LSB\_IDEAL} - 1\right| \tag{3.29}$$

where V_D or V_{D+1} is the converted analog value, the ideal LSB of V_{LSB_IDEAL} is Δ and $0 < D < 2^N - 2$. The expression of INL is defined as:

$$INL = \left|\left(V_D - V_{ZERO}\right) / V_{LSB\_IDEAL} - D\right| \tag{3.30}$$

where $0 < D < 2^N - 1$.

In the range of full-scale input (FSR), DNL and INL exhibit cyclical changes. The peak values appear every FSR/16, where the maximum deviation of the transfer curve affected by e_A and the ideal curve. With 12.1-bit accuracy, the maximum DNL and INL are both 1 LSB. Therefore, the resolution of the presented VPC with multisteps method can reach 16-bit in theory when the amplification accuracy is higher than 12.1-bit.

As mentioned above, the amplification error e_A is mainly contributed by components' mismatching and amplifiers' errors. In practical circuit design,

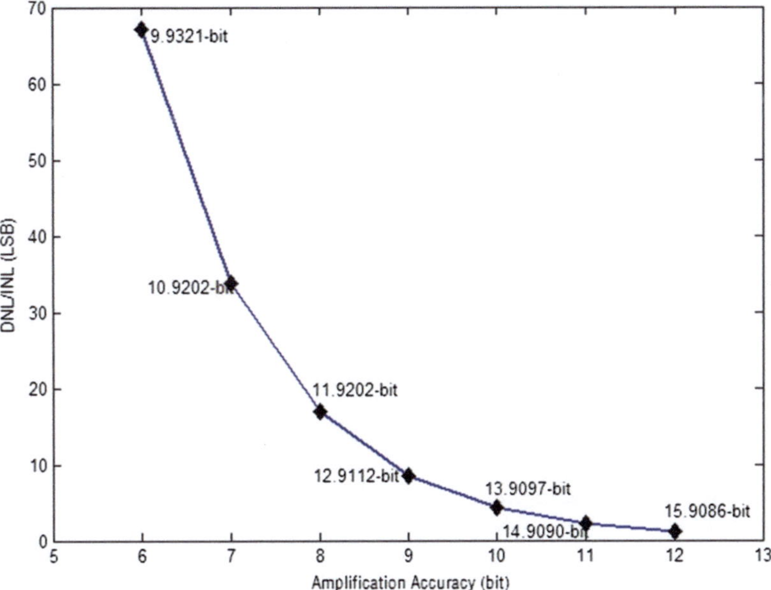

Fig. 3.47 The influence of amplification accuracy on VPC's resolution

switched-capacitor structure is applied for 2^4 times amplifier. In modern technologies, capacitor matching is good enough to obtain a full linearity specification up to 12-bit resolution without trimming [28]. For matching optimization, symmetry rule is applied in our design, and the capacitor devices, consisting of well-defined identical units, are placed in parallel or series. Assuming the ratio of C_A to $C_A^{'}$ is equal to 16 ideally, in order to achieve 12.1-bit amplification accuracy, the open-loop gain of OTA2 should be larger than 96.9 dB (about 70,239.7) [29]. In this design, a folded cascode structure with gain-booster is applied for OTA, and OTA's open-loop gain is larger than 100 dB under a ±0.6–1.8 voltage supply. Additionally, nonoverlapping clock and complementary switches have been utilized to avoid the charge injection effect.

Higher amplification error leads to lower resolution. As illustrated in Fig. 3.47, DNL and INL are changed from 1.06 LSB to 67.09 LSB with the amplification accuracy from 12-bit to 6-bit, which leads to the VPC's resolution of 15.9-bit to 9.9-bit.

There are still some errors such as finite gain error, switch errors from clock-through and charge injection, PSRR noise from supply, nonideal reference, and so forth. Thus, it may be impossible for the presented digitizer to achieve an ideal 16-bit resolution. If the amplification accuracy is lower than 8-bit, the VPC's resolution will be smaller than 11.9-bit as shown in Fig. 3.47. However, most nonideal effects are difficult to be predicted in prototype circuit design. Therefore, the cyclical 4-bit quantization operation can be performed four times for one complete conversion cycle.

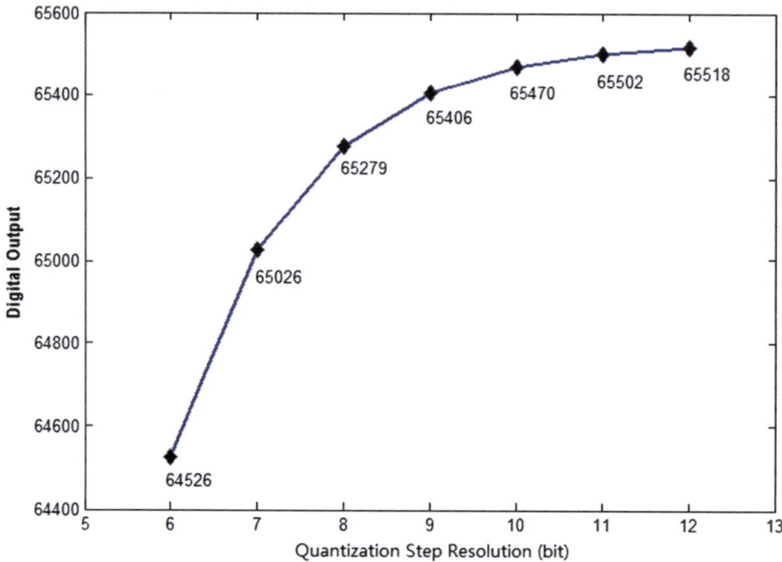

Fig. 3.48 The influence of quantization step error on output dynamic range. $e_B = 1/2^b$, where b is the resolution of quantization step

As sketched in Fig. 3.45, e_B changes the slope of the transfer curves. Assuming e_B is larger than 0, the influence of quantization step error on the output dynamic range is shown in Fig. 3.48. High quantization step error reduces the VPC's maximum output obviously. To the contrary, if $e_B < 0$, the quantization step error will cause output saturation and reduce the input dynamic range.

Additionally, there are some other error sources in the discussed VPC, such as the reference voltage drift or the power supply imbalance. These kinds of errors will make the transfer curve in Fig. 3.45 parallel shifted. It might affect the input dynamic range, but would not decrease the linearity and could be removed by postprocessing.

Output Structure and Update Rate

A pulses-formed data output is achieved by combining ϕ_A and ϕ_B as shown in Fig. 3.43. This single-line pulses-formed output structure is designed for short-distance data transmission. There are three kinds of pulses in one cycle, start-pulse (the width is 2 clock cycles), conversion-pulses (the width is 1 clock cycle), and borrow-pulses (width is 1/2 clock cycle). The interval time between two conversion-pulses (or the start-pulse and the first conversion-pulse) is from 2 to 17 clock cycles, which represents a 4-bit quantization value from 0000 to 1111. Every cycle has four conversion-pulses. Therefore, a 16-bit digital output code can be carried by the intervals in one complete conversion cycle. Borrow-pulse is used for self-calibration. When a borrow-pulse occurs in any conversion interval behind start-pulse or

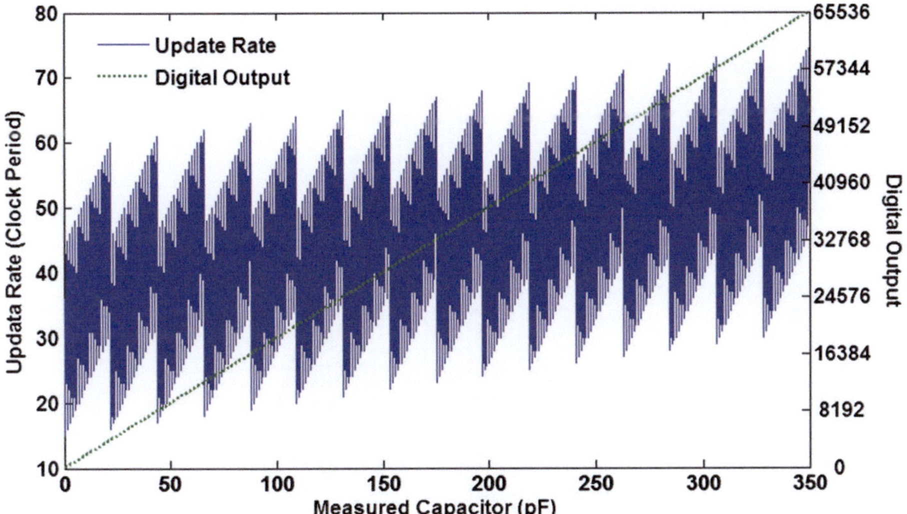

Fig. 3.49 Output and conversion time (updateing rate) of the VPC when used fo capacitive sensor

conversion-pulses, the previous interval should be corrected with minus 1 clock cycles. In this work, a new conversion operation begins immediately after the previous conversion as described in Fig. 3.43. Because the time interval of one quantization phase ranges from 2 to 17 clock cycles and the pulses between conversion phases occupy 7 clock cycles, one complete conversion cycle of the presented readout IC needs 15–75 clock cycles. In [30], in order to obtain a synchronized data output, the voltage–pulse converter is reset every 80 clock cycles. Since the conversion can be completed within 15–75 clock cycles (the update rate), the remaining 5–65 clock cycles are wasted. Therefore, compared to the output structure in [30], this design has a dynamic update rate distributed from 15 to 75 clock cycles instead of a fixed 80 clock cycles in the former version, which greatly improves the performance of update rate.

As is described above, the conversion time of four quantization phases in one complete cycle are d_1, d_2, d_3, and d_4, respectively. Thus, the total 0063onversion time is given as:

$$d_t = d_1 + d_2 + d_3 + d_4 + d_p \tag{3.31}$$

where d_p is the duration time of pulses in one cycle, whose value is 7 clock cycles. Because $d_1 \sim d_4$ takes 2–17 clock cycles, the update rate is not fixed, which is determined by the value of measured capacitance. Figure 3.49 shows the digital data output and conversion time of the presented capacitance-to-digital converter (CDC). In the range of full-scale, the conversion time spirals with the measured capacitance value increasing.

Assuming the input signal is uniformly distributed in magnitude, by statistically investigating the update time, the distribution of the data update time tends to be

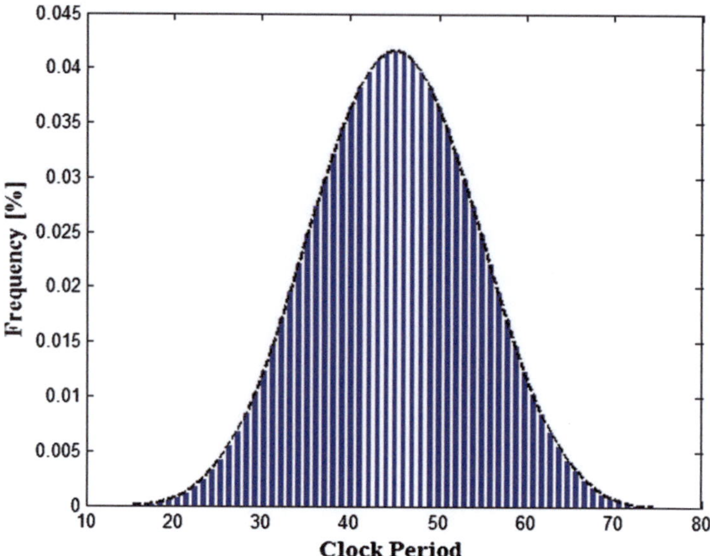

Fig. 3.50 Statistical results of update time with full-scale input

a normal distribution. The statistical result is illustrated in Fig. 3.50. The mean and the standard deviation of update rate are 45 clock cycles and 9.43 clock cycles, respectively.

3.4   A Capacitive Sensor Readout Circuit

Capacitive sensors array has attractive features of low energy consumption and simple structure. The capacitive sensors are widely used in wireless medical/health care systems. In a capacitive sensor, the capacitive elements, which are built with conductive sensing electrodes in a dielectric, convert nonelectrical quantities into capacitive quantities. However, there is a bottleneck for signal conditioning of these capacitive sensors array. Due to high parasitic capacitance or some contamination under uncertainty, absolute capacitance values of sensors may range from sub-pF up to hundreds of pF and may change very fast with sensed signals in some applications, such measurements should not be performed using low-cost sensor system. Therefore, a cost-effective signal conditioning solution for capacitive sensors array with features of fast update rate and wide capacitance measurement range is desirable.

Some previously reported results provide excellent solutions for capacitive sensor signal acquisition, which convert the capacitance into voltage, frequency, or pulse width modulation for further analysis and processing [4, 31–35]. These traditional capacitive sensor interfaces are usually composed of a switch matrix, a sigma-delta (Σ–Δ) converter, the standard data interface, and other modules. However, this type capacitive interface has low dynamic range. The measurement range is usually

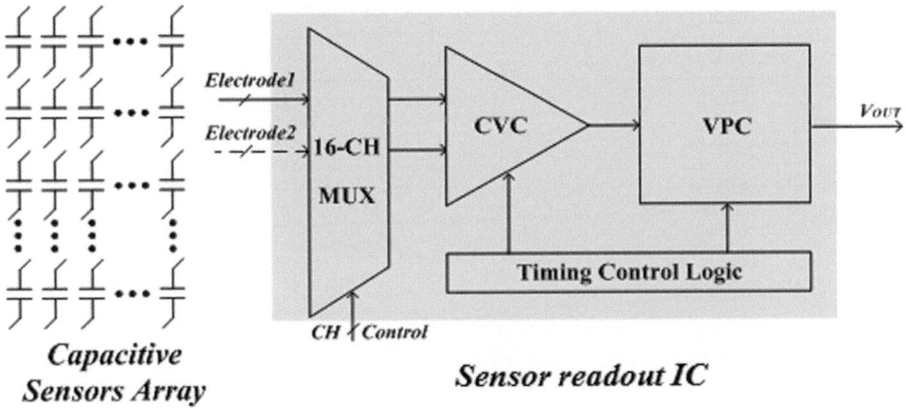

Fig. 3.51 Block diagram of the capacitive sensor readout IC

around tens of pF. Another type, named quasi-digital sensor interface, transforms the sensor variations into quasi-digital forms, including frequency, time period, duty cycle, etc. [33–35]. The quasi-digital type usually has wide input dynamic range (up to 300 pF), but suffers from low update rate (usually 10 or 100 ms for one channel), high power consumption, and low process consistency, which is not suitable for multisensors applications. These shortcomings limit the utilization of the commercial ICs in capacitive sensor array with wide capacitance measurement range and fast update rate.

Using the techniques presented in the previous subsections, a novel CMOS CDC with a 16-bit target resolution for capacitive biomedical sensors array readout can be implemented. It has wide linear input range (up to 350 pF) and short measurement time (no more than 0.75 ms per channel). This circuit consists of a 16-ch multiplexer (MUX), a CVC as shown in Sect. 3.2.1, and a voltage–pulse converter (VPC) as shown in Sect. 3.3.3. The block diagram of the entire sensor readout circuit is shown in Fig. 3.51.

The implemented capacitive sensor readout IC has been designed and fabricated in 0.18 μm 1P6M CMOS technology with a active area of 640×630 μm^2 (Fig. 3.52). The testing results show that the maximum absolute input capacitance is 350 pF with a dynamic measurement time (0.15–0.75 ms/ch) under a 100-kHz operating clock. The power consumption is 90 μA with ±0.9 V typical voltage supply.

To demonstrate the designed readout IC functionality, the input–output characteristic has been tested and depicted in Fig. 3.53. It converts the capacitance into pulses-formed single-line output with the operating clock of 48 kHz. The data output of 1011 0001 0100 1001 corresponds to 220 pF capacitance input, whereas 0100 0101 1110 0111 corresponds to 22 pF. It can be observed that there is a borrow-pulse in the conversion cycle of 22 pF capacitance. It means a wrong rollover occurs and the self-calibration circuit works to eliminate this conversion error.

Figure 3.54 shows the measurement for the presented CVC. After the reset pulse φ_R, the CVC output only needs 1.4 μs to be stable for further processing. The test was performed with a 330-pF capacitance input under a 100-kHz operation clock.

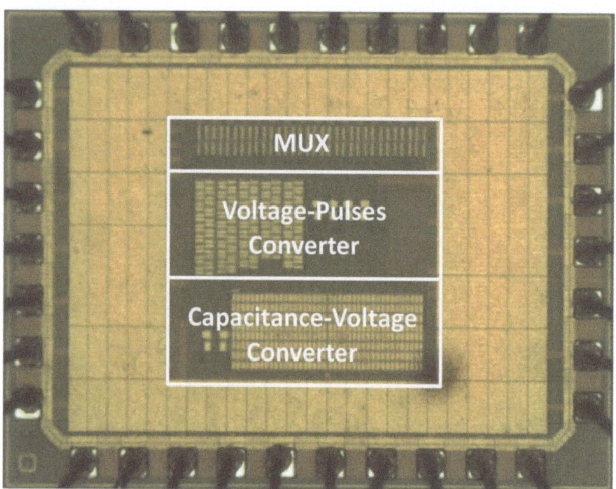

Fig. 3.52 Microphotograph of the capacitive sensor readout IC

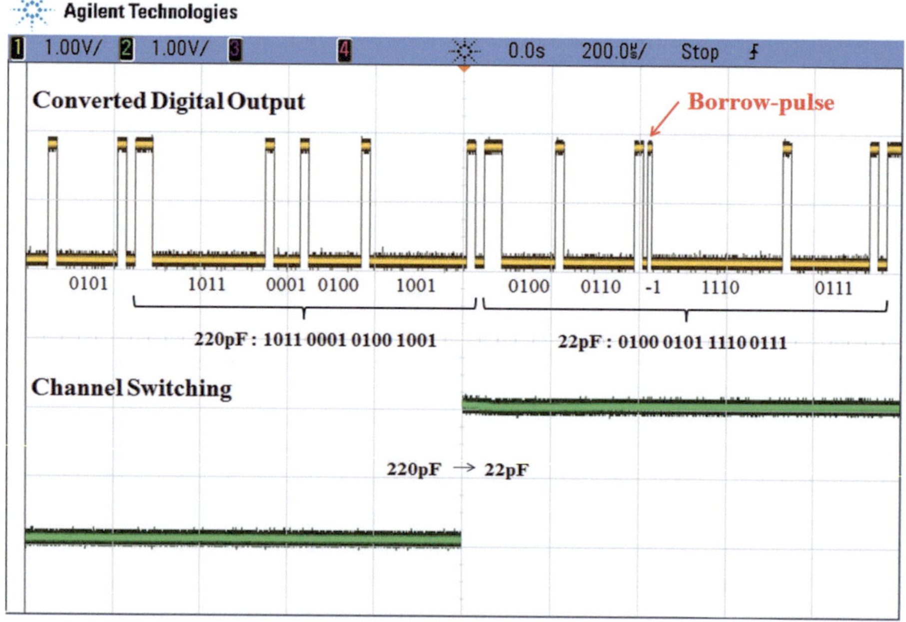

Fig. 3.53 Input–output characteristic of the design readout IC

The test for linearity and measurement range was performed by measuring the capacitance from 10 to 350 pF with a step of 20 pF. The transfer curve is illustrated in Fig. 3.55. The curve keeps linear in the full-scale range. The maximum value of input capacitance can reach to 350 pF. The operation clock was 100 kHz, corresponding to a dynamic update rate distributed from 0.15 to 0.75 ms/ch.

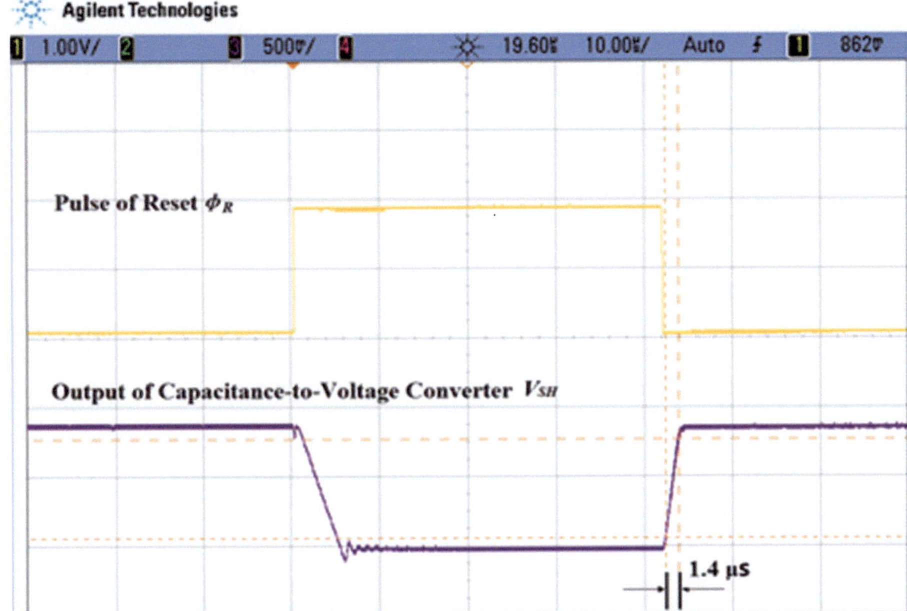

Fig. 3.54 Rising time in sample-and-hold operation

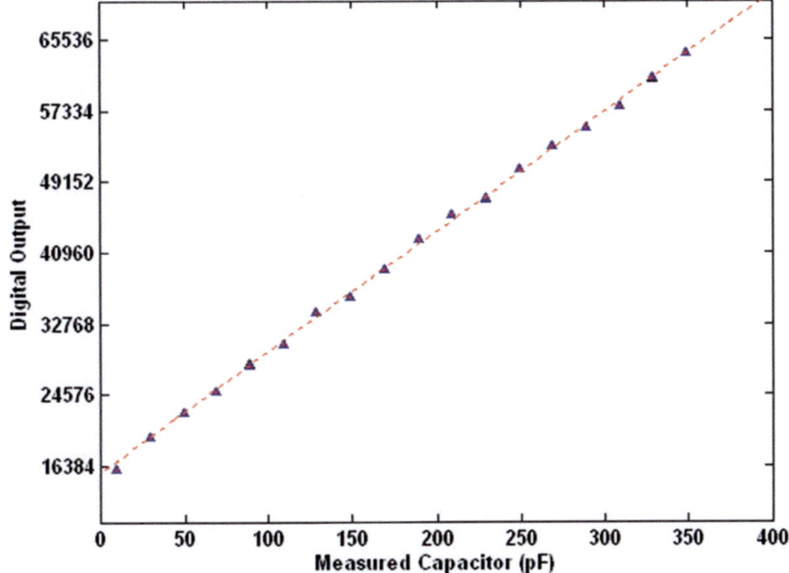

Fig. 3.55 Linearity and dynamic range measurement

Table 3.4 Capacitive sensor readout IC performance summary

Voltage (V)	±0.6–1.8
Supply current (µA)	85
Target resolution/ENOB (bit)	16/11.7
Measurement range (pF)	0–350
Channel	16
Measurement time/ch (ms)	0.75
Process (µm)	0.18

The ENOB of the presented voltage–pulse converter (VPC) was measured in [30]. The measurement results show that the VPC has an ENOB of 11.7 bits.

The performance of the capacitive sensor readout IC is summarized in Table 3.4. A remarkable performance has been achieved with the CVC and VPC techniques presented.

References

1. Honeywell, FSS Series low profile force sensor datasheet. http://sensing.honeywell.com.cn/?ci_id=145410, 2013.
2. Wong WM, Bautista J, Dekel R, et al. Feasibility and tolerability of transnasal/per-oral placement of the wireless pH capsule vs. traditional 24-h oesophageal pH monitoring—a randomized trial. Aliment Pharmacol Ther. 2005;21(2):155–63.
3. Kim H, Kim S, van Helleputt N, Artes A, Konijnenburg M, Huisken J, van Hoof C, Yazicioglu RF. A configurable and low-power mixed signal SoC for portable ECG monitoring applications. IEEE Trans Biomed Circuits Syst. http://ieeexplore.ieee.org/stamp/stamp.jsp?tp=&arnumber=6544283
4. Lee H-K, Chang S-II, Yoon E. A flexible polymer tactile sensor: fabrication and modular expandability for large area deployment. J Microelectromech Syst. 2006;15(6):1681–6.
5. Menolfi C, Huang Q. A low-noise CMOS instrumentation amplifier for thermoelectric infrared detectors. IEEE J Solid-State Circuits. 1997;32(7):968–76.
6. Makinwa KAA, Huijsing JH. A wind sensor with an integrated low offset instrumentation amplifier. In: ICECS. Sep, 2001;1505–8.
7. Witte JF, Huijsing JH, Makinwa KAA. A current-feedback instrumentation amplifier with 5 µV offset for bidirectional high-side current-sensing. IEEE J Solid-State Circuits. 2008; 43(12):2769–75.
8. Fan Q, Sebastiano F, Huijsing JH, Makinwa KAA. A 1.8 µW 60 nV/$\sqrt{\text{Hz}}$ capacitively-coupled chopper instrumentation amplifier in 65 nm CMOS for wireless sensor nodes. IEEE J Solid-State Circuits. 2011;46(7):1534–43.
9. Chan PK, Ng KA, Zhang XL. A CMOS chopper-stabilized differential difference amplifier for biomedical integrated circuits. In: The 2004 47th Midwest symposium on circuits and systems, 2004. MWSCAS Aug, 2004, Hiroshima. 2004;III-33–6.
10. Denison T, Consoer K, Santa W, Molnar G, Miesel K. A 2 µW, 95 nV/$\sqrt{\text{Hz}}$, chopper-stabilized instrumentation amplifier for chronic measurement of bio-potentials. In: IMTC. May, 2007;1–6.
11. Fan Q, Sebastiano F, Huijsing H, Makinwa K. A 2.1 µW area-efficient capacitively-coupled chopper instrumentation amplifier for ECG applications in 65 nm CMOS. In: ASSCC. Nov, 2010;1–4.
12. Sansen WMC. Analog design essentials. Berlin: Springer; 2006.
13. Enz CC, Temes GC. Circuit techniques for reducing the effects of op-amp imperfections: autozeroing, correlated double sampling, and chopper stabilization. Proc IEEE. 1996;84(11): 1584–614.

14. Kitchin C, Counts L. A designer's guide to instrument amplifiers. 3rd ed. Cambridge: Analog Devices Inc.; 2006.
15. van den Dool BJ, Huijsing JH. Indirect current feedback instrumentation amplifier with a common-mode input range that includes the negative rail. IEEE J Solid-State Circuits. 1993;28(7):743–9.
16. Toumazou C, Lidgey FJ, Haigh DG. Analogue IC design: the current-mode approach. London: Peter Peregrinus Ltd.; 1990.
17. Witte JF, Makinwa KA, Huijsing JH. A CMOS chopper offset-stabilized opamp. IEEE J Solid-State Circuits. 2007;42(7):1529–35.
18. Burt R, Zhang J. A micropower chopper-stabilized operational amplifier using a SC notch filter with synchronous integration inside the continuous-time signal path. IEEE J Solid-State Circuits. 2006;41(12):2729–36.
19. Kusuda Y. Auto correction feedback for ripple suppression in a chopper amplifier. IEEE J Solid-State Circuits. 2010;45(8):1436–45.
20. Kusuda Y. A 5.9nV/$\sqrt{\text{Hz}}$ chopper operational amplifier with 0.78μV maximum offset and 28.3nV/°C offset drift. In: ISSCC 2011. p. 242–3.
21. Sanduleanu MAT, Van Tuijl AJM, Wassenaar RF, Lammers MC, Wallinga H. A low noise, low residual offset, chopped amplifier for mixed level applications. In: IEEE international conference on electronics, circuits and systems 1998, Vol 2, Lisboa; 1998. p. 333–6.
22. Menolfi C, Huang Q. A fully integrated, untrimmed CMOS instrumentation amplifier with submicrovolt offset. IEEE J Solid-State Circuits. 1999;34(3):415–20.
23. Bakker A, Thiele K, Huijsing JH. A CMOS nested-chopper instrumentation amplifier with 100-nV offset. IEEE J Solid-State Circuits. 2000;35(12):1877–83.
24. Wu R, Makinwa KAA, Huijsing JH. A chopper current-feedback instrumentation amplifier with a 1 mHz 1/f noise corner and an AC-coupled ripple reduction loop. IEEE J Solid-State Circuits. 2009;44(12):3232–43.
25. Gerrish P, Herrmann E, Tyler L, Walsh K. A cyclic A/D converter that does not require ratio-matched components. IEEE J Solid-State Circuits. 1988;23(1):152–8.
26. Lee H. A 12 bit 600 kS/s digitally self-calibrated pipeline algorithmic ADC. In: IEEE 1993 symposium on VLSI circuits; 1993. p. 121–2.
27. Allen PE, Holberg DR. CMOS analog circuit design. 2nd ed. Oxford: Oxford University Press; 2002. p. 480–3.
28. van de Plassche R. CMOS integrated analog-to-digital and digital-to-analog converters. 2nd ed. Dordrecht: Kluwer Academic; 2003. p. xxxvii.
29. Franco S. Design with operational amplifiers and analog integrated circuits. 3rd ed. New York: McGraw-Hill; 2001. p. 23–5.
30. Zhang X, Chen H, Liu M, Zhang C, Wang Z. Sensor interface with single-line quasi-digital output for ligament balance measuring system. In: IEEE biomedical circuits and systems conference, San Diego; 2011.
31. AD7147A Datasheet. 2009. http://www.analog.com/static/imported-files/data_sheets/AD7147A.pdf
32. LDS6200 Family Datasheet. 2011. http://www.idt.com/document/dst/lds6200-family-datasheet-rev-05-june-2011
33. Heidary A, Meijer GCM. Features and design constraints for an optimized SC front-end circuit for capacitive sensors with a wide dynamic range. IEEE J Solid-State Circuits. 2008;43(7):1609–16.
34. UTI Datasheet. 2010. http://www.smartec-sensors.com/assets/files/pdf/sensors/SMTUTIN.PDF
35. Goes VD, Meijier CM. A novel low-cost and accurate multiple-purpose sensor interface with continuous autocalibration. In: IEEE instrumentation and measurement technology conference; 1996.

Chapter 4
WBAN Transceiver Design

4.1 Narrow Band Short Range Wireless Transceivers

The tremendous progress in wireless medical and health care applications in recent years, as well as the significant improvements in wireless communication and semiconductor technologies, led to the rapid development in the wireless body area networks (WBAN) technologies [1, 2], which can be used to connected the PBS and SIDs in the wireless medical/health care systems as shown in Chap. 2.

4.1.1 Frequency Bands for WBAN Transceivers

The IEEE 802.15.6 WBAN standard was released by the IEEE LAN/MAN standards committee for the short-range low-power WBAN operated on, in, or around the human body (but not limited to humans) in February, 2012 [3]. The standard physical (PHY) layer defines a narrow band (NB) mode compliant device (hub/node, corresponding to PBS/SID in the application systems) shall be able to support at least one of the following frequency bands: 402–405, 420–450, 863–870, 902–928, 950–958, 2,360–2,400, and 2,400–2,483.5 MHz. Before the 802.15.6 standard was released, IEEE 802.15.4/ZigBee low-rate wireless personal area network (LR-WPAN) standard was also widely used for WBAN devices [4]. The IEEE 802.15.4 standard PHY layer defines its operation on one of the three possible unlicensed frequency bands: 868, 902–928, and 2,400–2,483.5 MHz [5]. In some occasions, the below VHF band is used for WBAN, including 6.78 MHz, 13.56 MHz, 27.15 MHz, and 9–315 kHz for inductive link.

The frequency available for WBAN in 400 MHz UHF, 2.4 GHz ISM and UWB bands for different countries and areas are illustrated in Fig. 4.1 [6].

Note that in real applications, only the 400 MHz and 2.4 GHz bands are most commonly used for the wireless medical and health care applications, since the 400 MHz band signal has small through-body transmission loss, and the

Z. Wang et al., *CMOS IC Design for Wireless Medical and Health Care*,
DOI 10.1007/978-1-4614-9503-1_4, © Springer Science+Business Media New York 2014

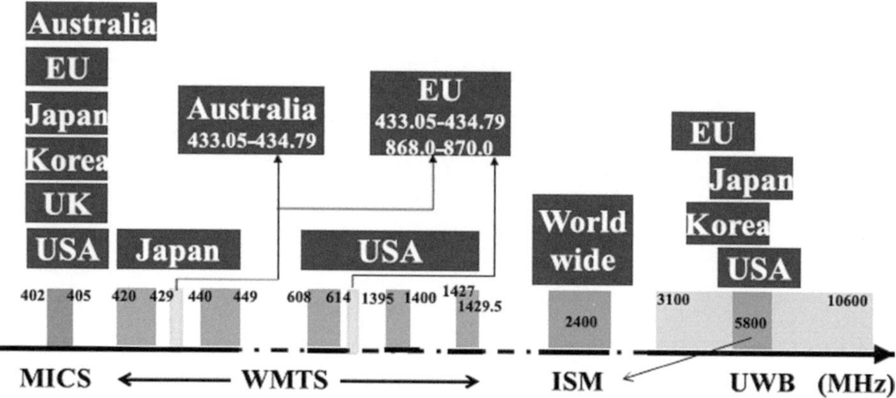

Fig. 4.1 Available frequency bands for WBAN, *Astrin et. al., Standardrization for Body Area Networks, IEICE Trans., Feb 2009* [6]

Table 4.1 Comparison of 400 MHz band and 2.4 GHz band for WBAN

	400 MHz	2.4 GHz
Through body loss	Small (+)	Large (−)
Bandwidth available	Small (−)	Large (+)
Antenna size required	Big (−)	Small (+)
Coexistence with other protocols	Less interference from other protocols (+)	Share the band with many other protocols (−)
Maximum allowed RF signal strength	Usually a few mW (−)	≥100 mW (+)

Note: (−) means negative impact, and (+) means positive impact

2.4 GHz band has large usable bandwidth and requires small antennas in WBAN applications.

There are three types of wireless communications in WBAN as mentioned below:

1. In the body: SID inside human body, PBS outside body
2. On the body: SID and PBS attached to the body
3. Around the body: SID attached to body, PBS near the body

Whether to use the 400 MHz band or the 2.4 GHz band depends on the real application conditions. To satisfy the miniaturization and low energy consumption requirements of the different WBAN applications, in-body and on/around-body SIDs (nodes) usually work on different communication frequencies. High frequency helps to reduce the antenna size, and the on/around-body nodes are usually designed in 2.4 GHz band to make their dimensions acceptable. However, the 2.4 GHz electromagnetic wave shows more propagation attenuation through the body tissue than the 400 MHz wave. In some applications, it is a good choice to choose 400 MHz band for in-body nodes to minimize the power consumption. Thanks to the high relative permittivity of the body tissue, which is about 30~60 in different tissues. The antenna of in-body nodes still can be designed in small dimensions. The comparison of the 400 MHz band and the 2.4 GHz band is shown in Table 4.1.

Previously reported wireless transceivers for WBAN PBS (hubs) only focused on the 400 MHz or the 2.4 GHz single band operation [7–12]. To make a WBAN hub that can work with multiple kinds of nodes in different bands in/on/around a certain person, the natural solution is to design a WBAN hub transceiver that covers the mainly used 400 MHz and 2.4 GHz WBAN bands, while to design the WBAN node transceivers at fixed frequency bands depending on the real applications.

These previously reported single band transceiver could not fulfill the above frequency band covering requirement. One possible solution is the software defined radio (SDR) architecture [13]. However, the SDR transceiver is usually designed for the continuous and wide band covering, and obviously not an optimal choice for the targeted WBAN hub transceiver, which only requires discontinuous and narrow bands covering. Actually, an SDR transceiver requires a local oscillate (LO) signal with drastically high tuning range (800–5,000 MHz) to shift signal frequency between quadrature IF signals and the wideband RF signals (400–2,500 MHz) directly, which is extremely power hungry and not suitable for WBAN applications.

Three WBAN transceivers/transmitters will be introduced in the following part of this chapter. The first two designs are dedicated for the SIDs in wireless medical/ health care system, whereas the third one is a multiband multimode half-duplex PBS transceiver for both IEEE 802.15.6 NB and ZigBee PHY standards, as well as for a dedicated protocol for the wireless endoscope capsule in the 402–434 MHz band with a high data rate of 3 Mbps for image data transmission [14].

4.1.2   Link Budget for Through-Body Communication

The communication channel for the through-body communication is the human body tissues. It is very difficult to characterize this communication channel precisely, for a few reasons:

- The 3-D geometry of the human body is quite complicated and varies a lot from person to person.
- Different body tissues exhibit quite different electrical parameters and vary for different frequency bands.
- The transmission loss is greatly correlated with the antenna characteristics and the impedance matching.
- It is also a difficult task to characterize the antenna characteristics inside the human body.

How to characterize the human body as a wireless communication channel falls out of the scope of this book. However, from the design experiences, it is suggested to do experiments to find the actual RF signal loss through the human body using the specific antenna under working conditions close to the real situations. For the preliminary experiments, the normal saline is a good substitute for quick measurement. Further experiments can be done on pigs, which have the similar tissue architecture as human beings as shown in Fig. 4.2.

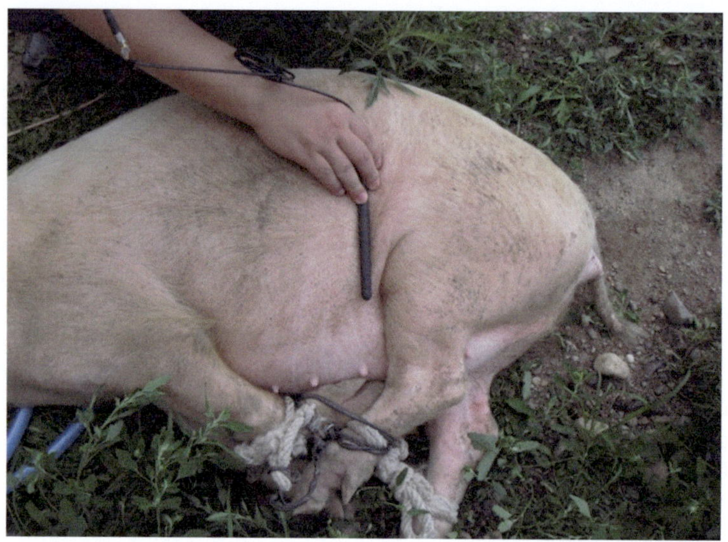

Fig. 4.2 Through-body communication experiment on a pig

The experiments from the authors' group found the following transmission path loss from the human gastrointestinal tract to the skin:

- 25 to 45 dB for the 400 MHz band
- 30 to 60 dB, sometimes up to 70 dB for the 2.4 GHz band

These numbers have been partially validated on the actual in-body wireless medical/health care devices.

With these results, the link budget for the through-body wireless communication can be derived as follows. The calculation is done for the data transmission from an SID (TX) inside human body to the PBS (RX) outside the body.

It can be easily found the received signal power at the input node of the PBS receiver is given by:

$$P_{RX}\big|_{dBm} = P_{TX}\big|_{dBm} + G_{TX}\big|_{dB} - P_{LOSS}\big|_{dB} + G_{RX}\big|_{dB} \tag{4.1}$$

where P_{RX} is the received signal power, and P_{TX} is the transmitted power from the SID transmitter, G_{TX} and G_{RX} are the transmitter and receiver antenna gain subtracted by mismatching loss, respectively, and P_{LOSS} is the transmission path loss.

SNR available at receiver IF output node is given by:

$$SNR_{RX}\big|_{dB} = P_{TX}\big|_{dBm} + G_{TX}\big|_{dB} - P_{LOSS}\big|_{dB} + G_{RX}\big|_{dB} - P_{Nin}\big|_{dBm} - NF_{RX}\big|_{dB} \tag{4.2}$$

where NF_{RX} is the PBS receiver overall noise figure, $P_{Nin}|_{dBm} = 10 \cdot \log(kTB)$, B is the PBS receiver bandwidth.

Assume that the PBS receiver has a digital demodulator, and the minimal acceptable *SNR* for demodulation is $SNR_{RX\min}$, then the minimum transmitted power from the SID transmitter is given by:

$$P_{TX\min}\big|_{dBm} = SNR_{RX\min}\big|_{dB} - G_{TX}\big|_{dB} + P_{LOSS}\big|_{dB} - G_{RX}\big|_{dB} + P_{Nin}\big|_{dBm} + NF_{RX}\big|_{dB} \quad (4.3)$$

If a 2 Mbps MSK link is calculated, and the PBS receiver has a zero-IF structure with $B = 3MHz$, $SNR_{RX\min} = 12dB$ for 10^{-3} BER at the RX side, $NF_{RX} = 4dB$, a huge $G_{TX} = -25dB$ due to SID antenna size limitation, $P_{LOSS} = 45dB$, $G_{RX} = 0dB$, then

$$P_{Nin}\big|_{dBm} = -174dBm + 10\log(3e6) = -109dBm$$

$$P_{TX\min} = 12 - (-25) + (45) - 0 - 109 + 4 = -23dBm$$

This means the SID transmitter needs to have an output signal level not less than $-23dBm$ so that the PBS receiver can correctly receive the data from the SID.

4.2   A 2.4 GHz SID Transmitter

In this section, the transmitter for miniature SIDs with burst data transmission will be discussed. As shown in Chap. 2, in wireless medical and health care SIDs with burst data transmission requirement, the constraints of the wireless transceiver are extremely different from those conventional wireless applications. First of all, the communication is highly asymmetric since the data flow is mostly transferred from inside to outside of human body. Second, high data transmission rate about several Mbps must be retained to transmit burst sensor data. Last and which is the most important, low power transceiver are typically required since the small size and low-capacity batteries are used. Due to the foregoing characteristics, low-power and high data rate transmitter has been a challenge to implement the wireless medical/health care system.

In addition to the requirements of the low power consumption and the high-reliable data rate, the higher integration level is also an issue for the small SIDs. Hence, various levels of system design hierarchy, from the modulation technique and the circuit architecture to the selection of the carrier frequency, must be explored to maximize the lifetime of the battery and minimize the size of the SIDs.

In low power transmitter, the constant amplitude FSK modulation techniques are generally selected to achieve the higher power efficiency using the nonlinear power amplifier [15]. However, for miniature SIDs using FSK modulation techniques, the smaller SID dimension requires the higher carrier frequency, a power-hungry frequency synthesizer is required to generate the desired frequency used in FSK modulation. In this section, the ASK modulation technique is used for its weak frequency dependency, a simple RF LC oscillator with an off-chip high-Q inductor is used as the carrier frequency generation circuits in order to acquire the higher power efficiency with the linear power amplifier, a pseudo-differential stacked class-A power amplifier is adopted.

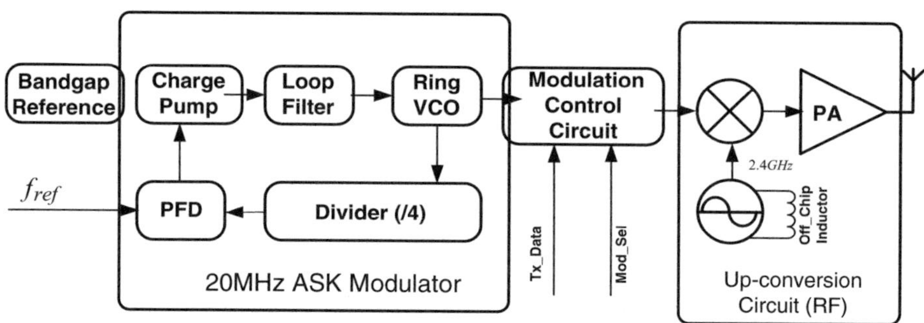

Fig. 4.3 ASK transmitter architecture

A 2.4 GHz ASK transmitter suitable for miniature wireless medical and health care SID with Mbps data rate will be presented in this section. The mixer-based frequency up-conversion transmitter architecture is employed to achieve high data rate. A pseudo-differential stacked class-A power amplifier using the current reused technique is proposed to save power consumption. The transmitter mainly includes two parts: a 20 MHz ASK modulator based on the constant amplitude phase-locked loop (PLL) and a direct up-conversion RF circuit. This design, implemented in 0.25 μm CMOS process, has achieved −23 dBm output power with the data rate of 1 Mbps and dissipates 3.17 mA current from a 2.5 V power supply.

4.2.1 Transmitter Architecture

In the traditional ASK transmitter architecture, the RF oscillator starts or dies under the control of the transmitted base-band data to implement the ASK modulation. In the low-power ASK transmitter, the startup time of RF oscillator is long, which seriously restrict the data rate of ASK system. Therefore, the traditional ASK transmitter is often used in low data rate wireless system. However, in wireless medical/ health care system, the requirements of high-quality burst sensor data demand to exploit the new transmitter architecture to achieve a high data transmission rate. Based on the mixer-based frequency up-conversion transmitter architecture, a high data rate ASK transmitter for wireless medical/health care applications is shown in Fig. 4.3. This ASK transmitter can be divided into two parts: the 20*MHz* ASK modulator and the direct up-conversion RF circuit. First, a low-frequency PLL with well-defined output amplitude is employed to generate the 20*MHz* carrier frequency. Then, under the control of the base-band data *Tx_Data* and the modulation mode selection *Mod_Sel*, the 20*MHz* ASK modulation signals can be achieved through the modulation control circuits. The up-conversion RF circuit up-converts the low-frequency ASK signal to the 2.4 GHz ISM band, then a micro-antenna transmits the modulation signal to the outside of human body. A temperature-independent and

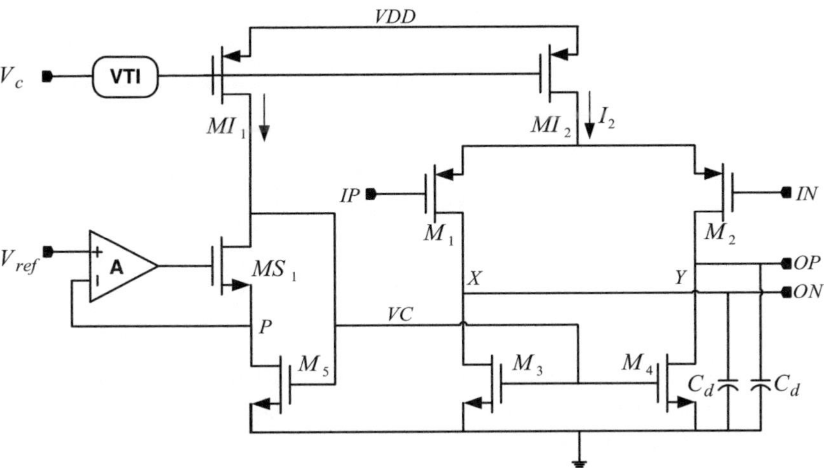

Fig. 4.4 The replica bias delay cell

high supply rejection reference is designed to provide the reference current and voltage for the ASK transmitter. In order to achieve the smaller dimension SID, almost all the building blocks are integrated besides a high-Q off-chip inductor.

4.2.2 Building Blocks

4.2.2.1 Low-Frequency Phase-Locked Loop (PLL)

A simple integer-N PLL is used to generate the low-frequency carrier. It includes a divide-by-4 asynchronous divider, a constant amplitude ring VCO, a rail-to-rail charge pump, a zero dead zone phase frequency detector (PFD), and a second-order loop filter (as shown in Fig. 4.3). When PLL is locked to the reference frequency of f_{ref}, in the output of ring VCO, an accurate frequency $4f_{ref}$ is achieved which acts as the low-frequency carrier.

   In low-frequency carrier generation circuit, the key block is the ring VCO with the well-defined output amplitude. In general, according to switching behavior, implementations of ring VCO can be categorized into two types: fixed swing and full swing. The full swing ring VCO is not suitable to be used in wireless capsule endoscope system for its high dynamic power consumption. So in this design, the fixed swing ring VCO using the replica bias technique is explored [16]. This VCO includes three delay stages and each delay cell is realized by the source-coupled circuit with PMOS differential input devices and NMOS triode-region load devices. The benefits of using a fully differential delay cell are its good power supply rejection and process variation immunity. The schematic diagram of the replica bias delay cell is shown in Fig. 4.4. The replica bias circuits include a feedback

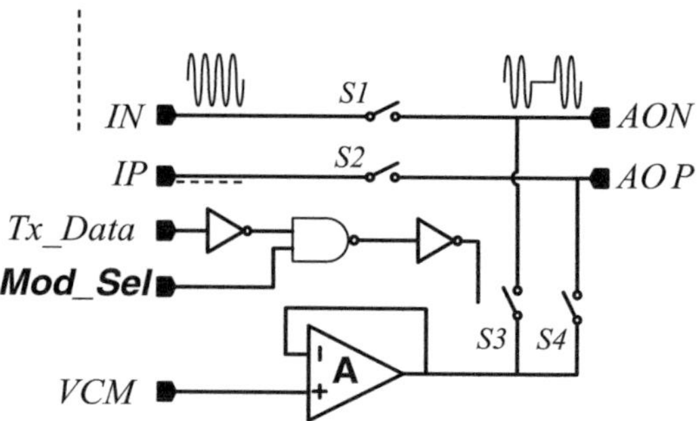

Fig. 4.5 Modulation control circuits

amplifier A, a voltage-controlled PMOS current transistor M_{I1}, a source follower M_{S1} and a triode-region transistor M_5. M_{I2} and $M_1 \sim M_4$ constitute the unit delay stage. The building block *VTI* is a high linearity voltage-to-current converter. The extra capacitors C_d are added at the output nodes to achieve the desired delay for the given application. If the loop gain is sufficiently large, the drain voltage of M_5 $V_P \approx V_{ref}$, the small V_{ref} will force M_5 to perform as a linear resistor. Once M_3 and M_4 are identical to M_5 and I_2 is identical to I_1, the on-resistance of M_3 and M_4 is equal to that of M_5, then the output nodes voltage V_X and V_Y vary from 0 to V_{ref} as M_1 and M_2 steer the tail current I_2 to one side or the other. Hence, using the replica bias technique, the well-defined output amplitude is achieved which is equal to the reference voltage V_{ref}. With the invariable output amplitude and load capacitor C_d, the delay of unit delay stage t_{delay} can be approximated as:

$$t_{delay} = \frac{C_d \cdot V_{ref}}{I_2} \tag{4.4}$$

Equation 4.4 indicates t_{delay} is the monotonic descent function of the tail current I_2. As mentioned earlier, *VTI* will ensure I_2 to be proportional to the control voltage V_c. Therefore, t_{delay} is inversely proportional to V_c, it will ensure the linear monotonicity between the frequency of ring VCO and the control voltage V_c.

4.2.2.2 Modulation Control Circuits

Modulation control circuits are the interface between the low-frequency PLL and the RF up-conversion circuits. The schematic diagram is depicted in Fig. 4.5. *Mod_Sel* is used to select the modulation mode. When *Mod_Sel* is "0," S1 and S2 are "ON", and S3 and S4 are "OFF", modulation control circuits will be bypassed and the input signal is directly shown in output nodes. When *Mod_Sel* is "1," modulation control circuits perform as a ASK modulator.

If the transmitted data *Tx_Data* = 1, S1 and S2 are "ON", and S3 and S4 are "OFF", the low-frequency carrier directly transfers to the output. If *Tx_Data* = 0, S1 and S2 are "OFF", and S3 and S4 are "ON", the output voltage is equal to the common-mode level *VCM* of the input node, which ensure the fast transition time when *Tx_Data* changes from "0" to "1."

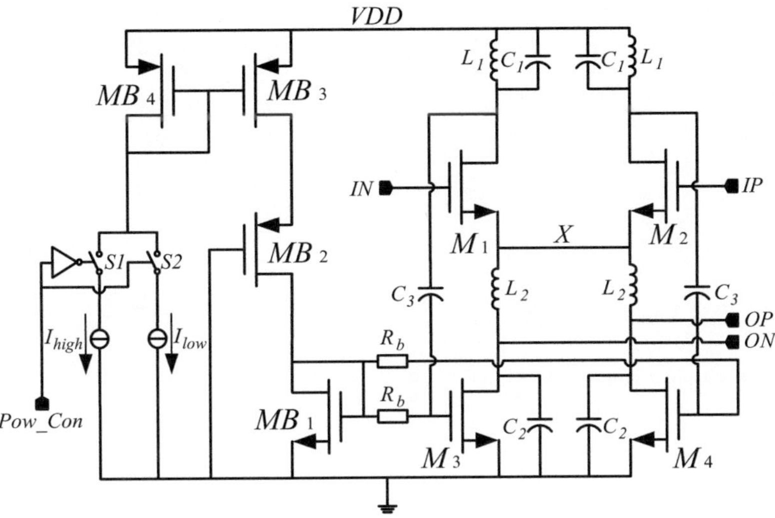

Fig. 4.6 The differential stacked class-A PA

4.2.2.3   Up-Conversion RF Circuits

Up-conversion RF circuits include three parts: a 2.4 GHz oscillator with the high-Q off-chip inductor, an up-conversion mixer with inductor load and a pseudo-differential stacked class-A PA. The low-frequency ASK signal is firstly up-converted to 2.4 GHz frequency band through the up-conversion mixer, then the stacked PA amplifies and transmits the modulated signal. Since the ASK modulation signal is insensitive to the frequency variation, the open-loop oscillator with coarse tuning is used as LO generation for low power consumption application.

In wireless capsule endoscope system, the maximum output power is less than 0 dBm, which allows the current-reuse technique in the design of PA. The schematic diagram of the proposed stacked PA is shown in Fig. 4.6. M_1, M_2, L_1 and C_1 constitute the first-stage amplifier, it is stacked on the output stage that consists of M_3, M_4, L_2 and C_2. The capacitor C_3 couples the output of the first stage to the input of the output stage. The current of the output stage is reused by the first-stage amplifier which is used to save power. Voltage node X provides ac ground which avoids the interference each other between two amplifier stages. M_{B1}~M_{B4} and S_1 & S_2 constitute the current bias circuits. *Pow_Con* is used to control the output power: when *Pow_Con*=1, S_2 is *ON* and the lower current I_{low} infuses the bias circuit, so the low output power will be transmitted; when *Pow_Con*=0, the higher current I_{high} is infused, and the high output power will be transmitted.

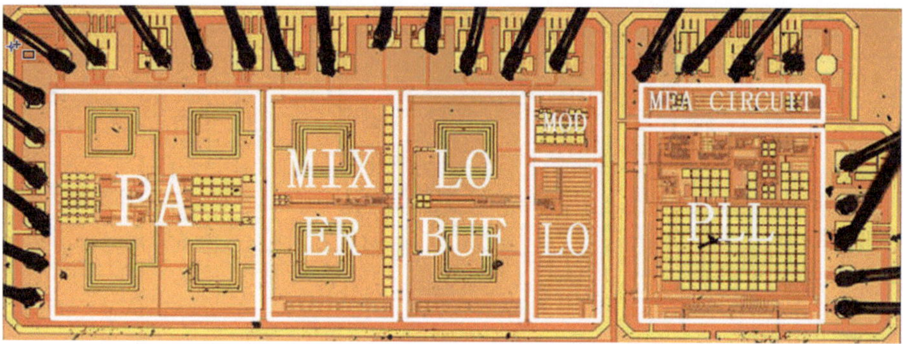

Fig. 4.7 Microphotograph of ASK transmitter

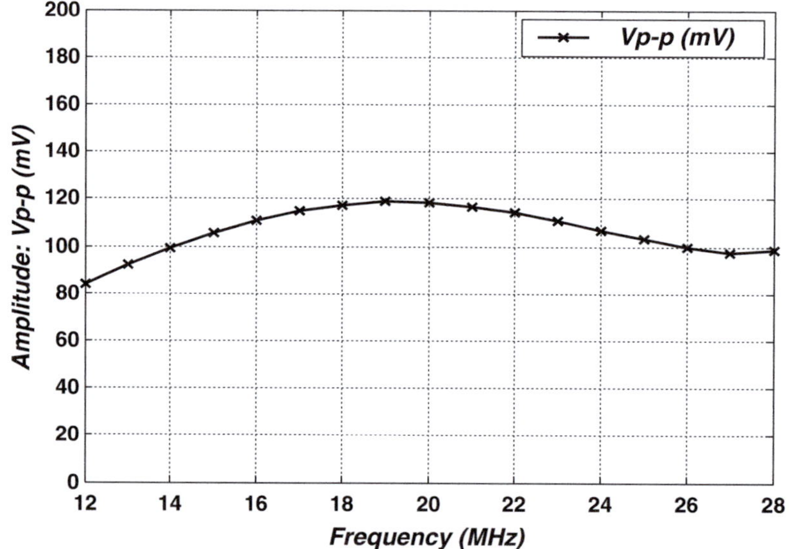

Fig. 4.8 Measured signal amplitude of PLL

4.2.3   Measurement Results

To verify the performance of the designed ASK transmitter, the proposed circuit has been fabricated in 2P6M 0.25 µm CMOS process. Figure 4.7 shows the microphotograph of the ASK transmitter, the die size is 1170×3097 µm². Except one discrete inductor, all the components are integrated in IC. For measurement convenience, the PA output directly connects to a 50 Ω load which acts as the antenna.

The measured signal peak-to-peak amplitude of low-frequency PLL is shown in Fig. 4.8. The maximum signal amplitude is 119 mV when the PLL is locked at

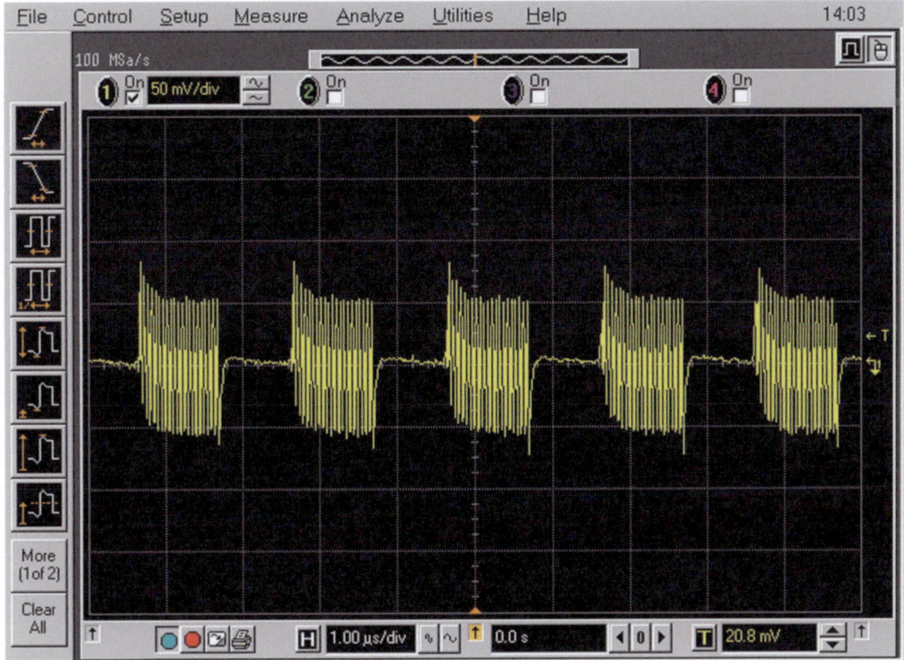

Fig. 4.9 Measured 20 MHz ASK signal with 1 Mbps data

19.5 MHz and the minimum signal amplitude is 84.5 mV when the PLL is locked
at 12 MHz. The measured PLL can be tuned between 6.5 and 36 MHz. Figure 4.9
shows the measured 20 MHz ASK signal with 1 Mbps input data.

Connecting the PA output to the vector signal analyzers, the modulated ASK
signal and the demodulated signal can be measured. The ASK modulation signal
spectrum with 1 Mbps data rate is shown in Fig. 4.10a, the output power is
−23.217 dBm with the 2.4 GHz center frequency. Figure 4.10b shows the demodulated signal where the input data rate is 1 Mbps, the current consumption is roughly
3.17 mA with the 2.5 V power supply.

Table 4.2 summarizes the measurement results of the designed ASK transmitter.
The proposed transmitter has higher data rate, higher integration level, higher carrier frequency, and lower energy consumption per bit.

In summary, a fully integrated ASK transmitter for miniature wireless medical/
health care SIDs with a high transmission data rate is presented in this section. The
low-frequency carrier with the well-defined amplitude is implemented using replica
bias technique. The pseudo-differential class-A PA with the current reused technique is used to save power. The transmitter works at 2.4 GHz frequency band and
is realized using the up-conversion technique. With 1 Mbps transmitted data,
−23.217 dBm output power can be achieved and only 3.17 mA current is dissipated
with 2.5 V power supply.

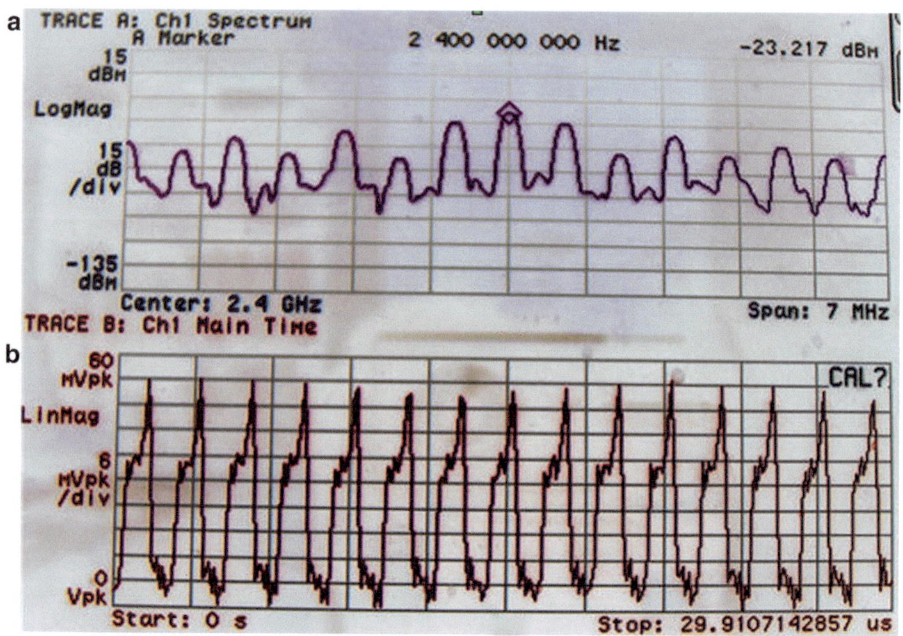

Fig. 4.10 (**a**) Modulated output ASK spectrum @ 1 Mbps, (**b**) ASK demodulation @ 1 Mbps

Table 4.2 2.4 GHz ASK transmitter performance summary

Supply voltage	2.5 V
Data rate	1 Mbps
Carrier frequency	2.4 GHz
Current consumption	3.17 mA
Energy consumption	7.925 nJ/bib
Output power	−23.217 dBm
Technology (CMOS)	0.25 μm
Chip area	3.62 mm^2

4.3 A 400 MHz 3 Mbps SID Transceiver

In this section, a design example of a 400 MHz transceiver designed for implantable wireless medical devices will be discussed to illustrate some design techniques that can be used for ULP transceivers with the constraints in the implantable medical applications. Note that the 400 MHz band is chosen for with the trade-off between through-body transmission loss and the antenna size.

4.3.1 Transceiver Architecture

The power consumption is the key issue for this transceiver. The overall structure of the transceiver used in this design is shown in Fig. 4.11. MSK modulation has been

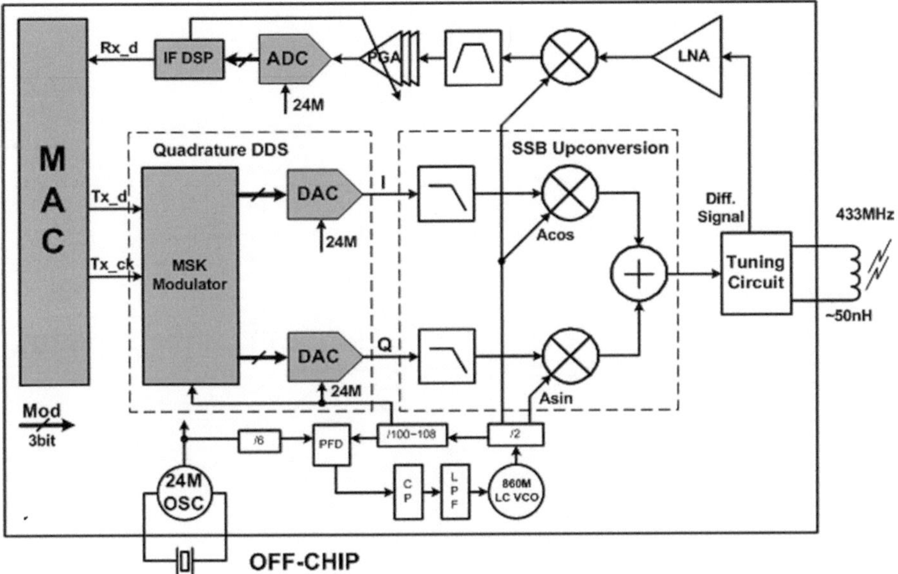

Fig. 4.11   400 MHz transceiver architecture

chosen for the transmitter, since MSK is a constant-envelope modulation, which can
help to alleviate the design requirement on the hub receiver. A high data rate of
3 Mbps is chosen such that the transmitter will be in a burst-mode and the average power
consumption of the transmitter will be quite low. The receiver takes a 64 kbps OOK
modulation for circuit simplification. Since the receiver is turned on very occasionally,
the transmitter will consume most of the system energy. Consequently, in this design,
the effort of power reduction has been mainly paid to the transmitter.

The transceiver works at the 400 MHz frequency band. A PLL frequency synthesizer is implemented on-chip to provide the quadrature LO signals for the transmitter
and the single phase LO signal for the receiver. The active circuit of a 24 MHz
crystal oscillator has been implemented to provide the reference clock for the PLL
and the system clock for the digital circuit.

As shown in Fig. 4.11, the MSK transmitter is composed of a quadrature direct
digital synthesizer (DDS) which converts the transmit data into the zero-IF analog
MSK baseband signal and a single sideband (SSB) up-converter which converts the
IF signal into the 400 MHz frequency band. The DDS consists of a digital MSK
modulator and a quadrature digital-to-analog converter (DAC) pair. The SSB up-
converter is mainly a quadrature up-mixer with the preceding low-pass anti-alias-
ing filter. The OOK receiver is composed of the low-noise amplifier (LNA) for RF
signal amplification, the down mixer for frequency down shifting, the band-pass
filter to suppress the out-of-band disturbance, the cascading programmable gain
amplifier (PGA) gain stages for IF signal amplification, the 3-bit analog-to-digital
converter (ADC) for quantization, and the IF DSP that performs the OOK
demodulation.

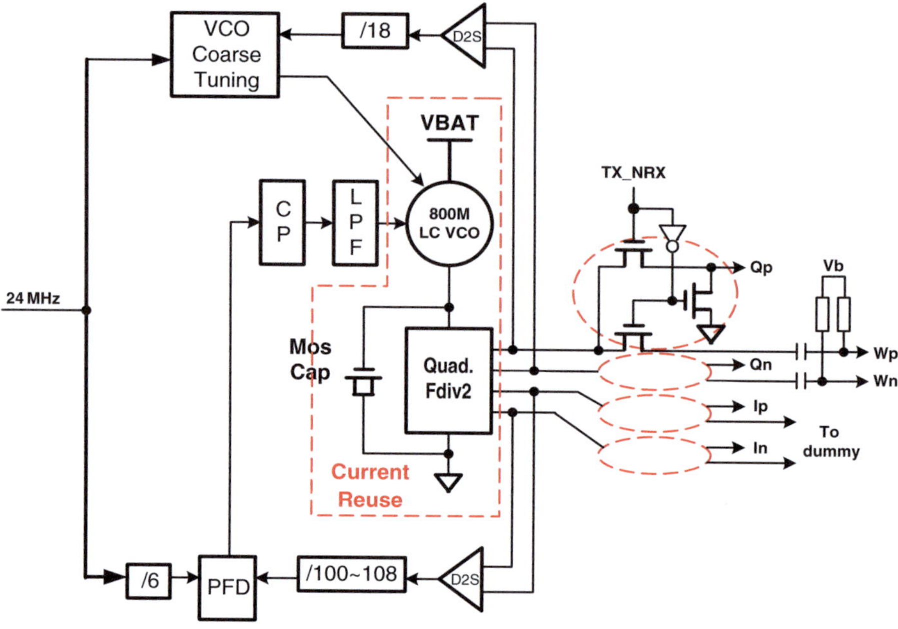

Fig. 4.12 Quadrature LO

In this design, all the power supply voltages are generated by on-chip linear regulators, as the switch regulator using inductors is not a good choice due to the number of external components and the consideration of EMI. Taking this in mind, the effort to lower the circuit power is equivalent to lower the circuit current. For this reason, current reusing techniques have been greatly adopted in the transceiver circuit. The current reusing techniques are mainly applied to the frequency synthesizer and the transmitter.

4.3.2 ULP Circuit Design Techniques

Figure 4.12 shows the structure of the frequency synthesizer. The VCO is designed to run at ~800 MHz to generate quadrature phase local oscillation signals. In this synthesizer, the quadratic frequency divider shares the same DC path as shown in Fig. 4.12 [17]. A classical PLL locks the VCO frequency. The PLL's divider is programmable, giving the SoC the capability of frequency hopping. The VCO has a coarse tuning circuit which helps to calibrate its center frequency automatically. Both the VCO tuning circuit and the PFD takes the reference frequency from the on-chip 24 MHz crystal oscillator.

The structure of the transmitter is shown in Fig. 4.13. In this transmitter, the MSK modulator receives the data stream from the main controller, transforms it into

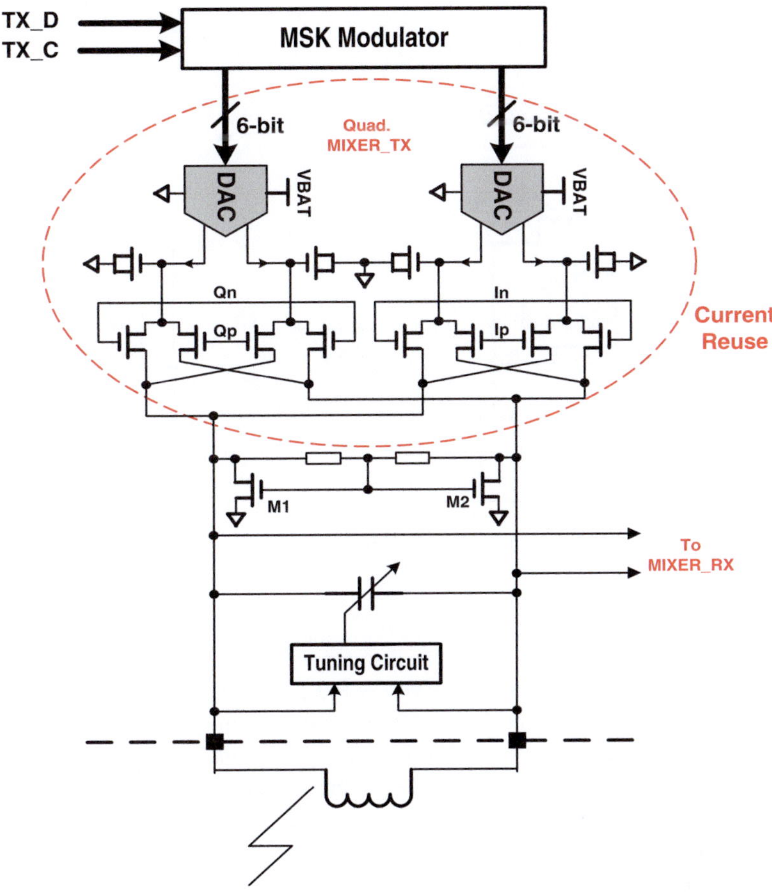

Fig. 4.13 Transmitter circuit with current reusing

zero-IF baseband waveforms, and then sends the parallel baseband data to the
DACs. There are two key points in this transmitter structures. First, the DCs of the two
DACs are reused by the quadrature mixer (M1 and M2 are used to set the DC path).
Second, there is no traditional power amplifier in this transmitter, and a coil which
serves as the RF energy emitting component is directly connected to the mixer. This
specific structure has been proven effective in the special application environment.

The transceiver uses a simple coil as the antenna. And the transmitter and the
receiver share an automatic tuning network. Note that in this specific application, it
is really difficult to achieve good antenna matching for the implanted device with a
traditional antenna, since the surrounding environment affects the antenna characteristic a lot, and it is quite difficult to characterize antenna's surrounding environment. In this design, the coil antenna can be viewed as an inductor as shown in
Figs. 4.13 and 4.14. C_{tune} is calibrated automatically so that the RF port achieves
resonance. There would be no traditional antenna in this design, and therefore there
is no need to do traditional antenna matching for this system.

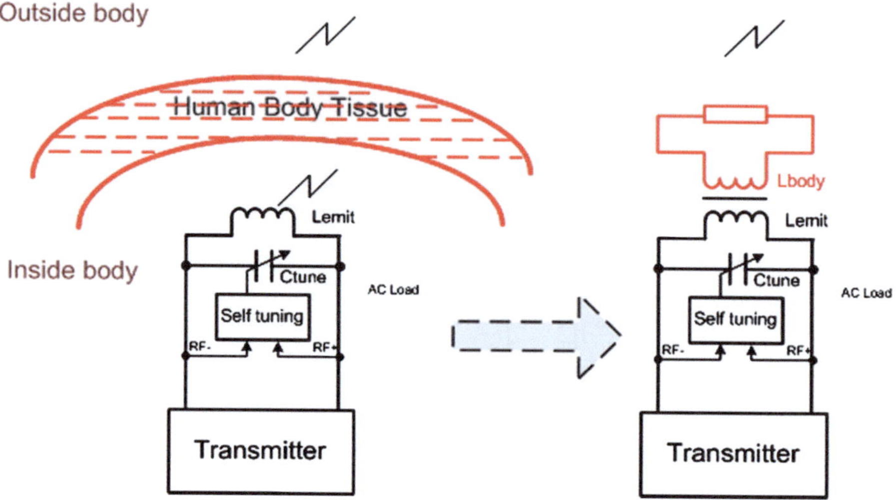

Fig. 4.14 Virtual transformer for through-body RF signal transmission

Actually, in this design a virtual transformer works as the antenna as illustrated in Fig. 4.14. Inductor L_{emit} actually serves as the primary coil emit, and the human body serves as the secondary coil. Of course, the transformer has very low coupling, which brings the benefit that the transmitter sees very steady load, and this helps to ease the circuit design work. On the other hand, the transmitting loss is quite high due to the low coupling effect, and this can be managed by set the RF AC level flowing through L_{emit}. Our experience is that if inductor L_{emit} has an RF AC of 10 mA (peak to peak), the external data recorder antenna can receive >−75 dBm RF signal from outside the human body, which is adequate for data demodulation.

4.3.3 Measurement Results

The ultra-low-power transceiver was fabricated in 0.18-μm 1P6M CMOS process.

The prototype chip is shown in Fig. 4.15. The bit rate of TX circuits is 3 Mbps and the power consumption is 3.9 mW, whereas the bit rate of RX circuits is 64 kbps and the power consumption is 12 mW.

To measure the fabricated transceiver, a capsule endoscope prototype with the transceiver PCB is encapsulated and put into a glass beaker (diameter 30 cm) filled with normal saline to emulate the real working environment as shown in Fig. 4.16.

The emitted MSK signal from the prototype capsule is then measured using a dipole antenna as the external receiving device. The received signal power by the external device can reach ~−55 dBm, which is far adequate for external receiving if the external data logger has a receiving sensitivity of −90 dBm.

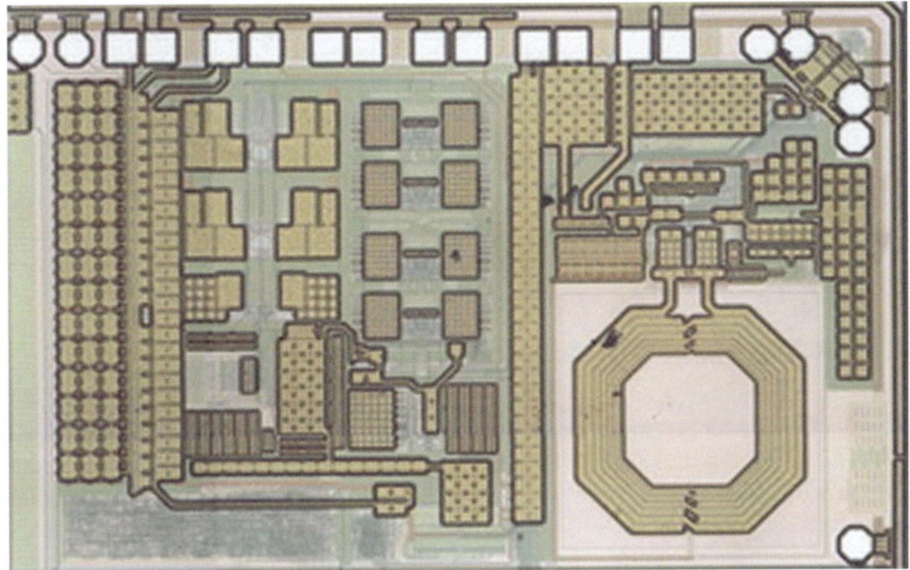

Fig. 4.15 Microphotograph of 400 MHz transceiver

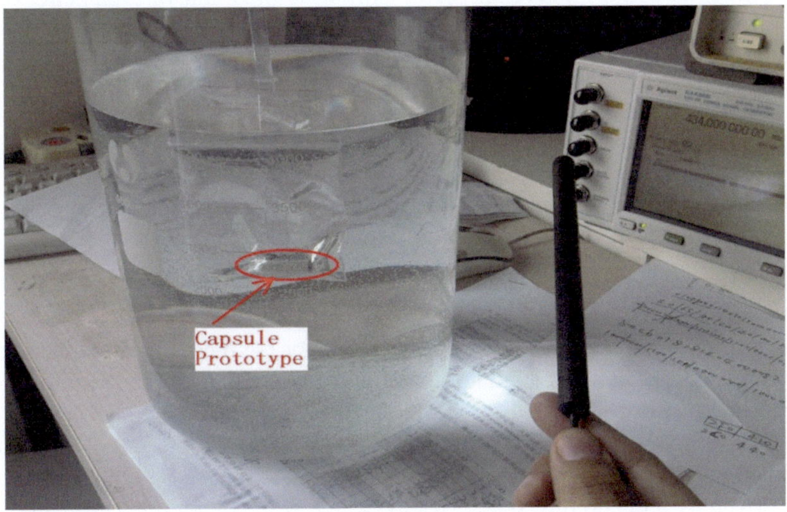

Fig. 4.16 Capsule endoscope prototype with designed 400 MHz transceiver in emulated environment

The performance of the implemented ultra-low-power 400 MHz transceiver is summarized in Table 4.3. The transmitter has a transmission efficiency of 1.3 nJ/bit, which makes it quite suitable for the implantable wireless medical applications.

Table 4.3 Performance of 400 MHz IMD transceiver

		Type of RF link	Bidirectional
TX		Bit rate	3 Mbps
		Modulation type	MSK
		Power consumption	3.9 mW
RX		Bit rate	64 kbps
		Modulation type	OOK
		Power consumption	12 mW
Technology			0.18 μm CMOS

4.4 A Multiband Multimode PBS Transceiver

This section presents a dual-band multimode half-duplex transceiver [18] for both IEEE 802.15.6 NB and ZigBee PHY standards, as well as for a dedicated protocol for the wireless endoscope capsule in the 402–434 MHz band with a high data rate of 3 Mbps for image data transmission [14]. It involves a novel reconfigurable sliding-IF transceiver architecture, which covers the 400 MHz and 2.4 GHz frequency bands without using the high-tuning range frequency synthesizer. The designed dual-band transceiver deploys a phase-locked loop (PLL) frequency synthesizer with only 21 % tuning range (1,608–1,988 MHz) to cover these bands. The implemented dual-band multimode transceiver exhibits comparable or even better performance in terms of noise, receiver sensitivity, phase noise, power consumption, and even die area compared to those transceivers reported in [7–12] for only a single band operation.

4.4.1 Reconfigurable Architecture

4.4.1.1 Transceiver Architecture

The sliding-IF architecture is an excellent option for the modern transceiver design. It shifts the RF signal into the analog baseband (ABB) signal with twice frequency conversions. As illustrated in Fig. 4.17, in the RX path, the received RF signal is first converted to the IF signal by a simple mixer using a single phase LO signal (f_{LO}), which is the VCO's direct output, and then converted to the ABB with the quadrature mixer driven by a quadrature signal (f_{LO_D}), which is the divide-by-2^n (n can be 1, 2 or 3) version of f_{LO}. The sliding-IF transceiver acts as a zero-IF transceiver if the ABB signal is centered at DC. Compared to the traditional zero-IF architecture, this architecture does not require the LO frequency as high as twice of the RF and thus widely used in low-power applications designed in the 0.13–0.18 μm low-cost CMOS process [9, 19].

Figure 4.18 shows the architecture of the proposed transceiver, it consists of a receiver (RX), a transmitter (TX), a frequency synthesizer with a LO distribution unit,

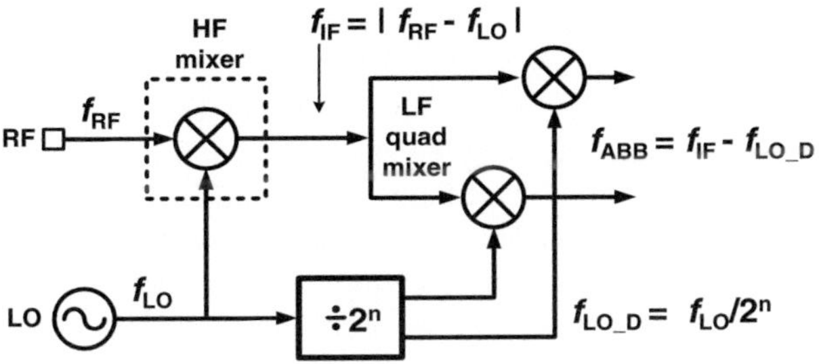

Fig. 4.17 Frequency conversions of the sliding-IF receiver

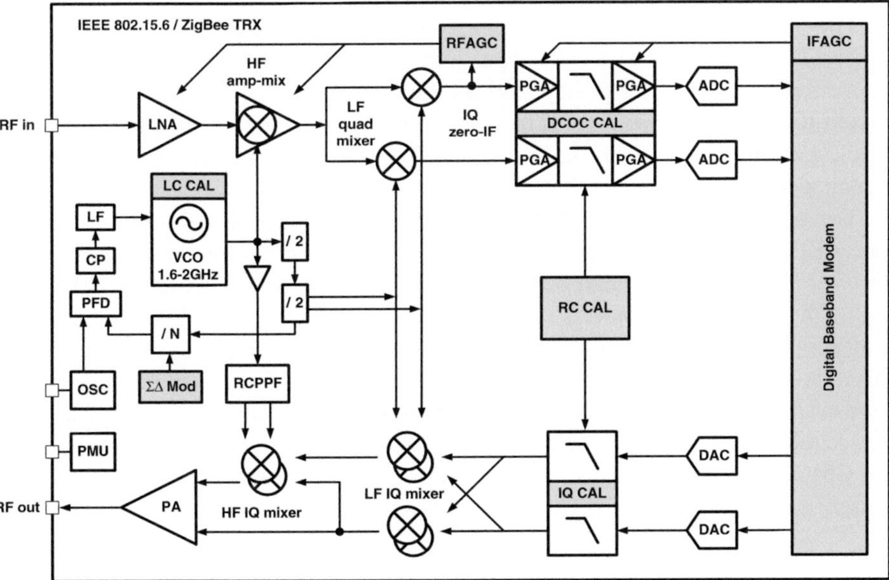

Fig. 4.18 Reconfigurable sliding-IF transceiver architecture

a digital baseband (DBB) modem for control and testing, and some auxiliary blocks such as the power management unit (PMU) and the on-chip oscillator (OSC). Compared to the classic sliding-IF transceiver discussed above, the proposed transceiver has a reconfigurable architecture, which merges the sliding-IF and zero-IF architectures together. Because there are different design considerations for RX and TX, the RX and TX reconfigurability is achieved in different ways as discussed in details below.

RX Reconfiguration

Noise performance is the major concern in the RX design, so it is important to avoid using signal switches, which introduces the insertion loss and declines the noise figure (NF).

The simple structure and low-noise circuits are preferred in the RX front-end design. The proposed RX front-end consists of an LNA, a reconfigurable high-frequency (HF) amplifier-mixer (amp-mix) and a low-frequency (LF) quadrature mixer. The HF amp-mix's LO can either be a single phase LO (f_{LO}) for double conversions or a DC signal for single conversion. The LF quadrature mixer LO f_{LO_D} frequency is $1/2^n$ of f_{LO} where the value of n depends on the frequency band selection. Therefore, the entire front-end is reconfigurable for receiving dual-band RF signals. (1) When the HF amp-mix acts as a simple mixer like the dash-boxed mixer in Fig. 4.17, the circuit serves as a sliding-IF receiver, and the 2.4 GHz RF input is converted to in-phase and quadrature (IQ) ABB signal in two steps. (2) When the HF amp-mix is reconfigured as an amplifier with a DC signal as its LO input, the 400 MHz RF input signals are directly converted to IQ ABB by mixing with f_{LO_D}.

The image (IM) problem might be a drawback when the RX is configured to the sliding-IF mode. Signals in the upper and lower band of the LO signal are both converted into the IF frequency, and the desired RF signal and the IM signal are mixed together in IF. A careful frequency plan can help to reduce the IM power level, and this problem can be further resolved by inserting RF filters before the nonquadrature mixer.

The ABB signal is chosen to be centered at DC in the RX, because the zero-IF-like ABB shows more advantages than the low-IF configuration in this multimode receiver. Note that the signal bandwidth widely varies from 200 kHz to 3 MHz to fulfill the IEEE 802.15.6 NB, ZigBee and a dedicated protocol for the wireless endoscope capsule, and thus a bandwidth reconfigurable ABB filter is required. One possible solution is to use large programmable arrays of resistors and capacitors. However, to maintain a good matching performance in such arrays for the strict image rejection ratio (IRR), requirement in low-IF receiver is extremely challenging for CMOS design. In contrast, the zero-IF receiver adopted in this design does not suffer from this problem since its IRR requirement is quite relaxed.

TX Reconfiguration

The dual-band TX frequency conversion mechanisms are similar to that of RX, but in a reversed direction. However, the TX circuit stature is quite different from what is used in RX due to a much severe IM problem when configured in the sliding-IF mode. The undesired IM sideband generated in the up-conversion using single phase LO's cannot be suppressed to fulfill the radio emission regulations if there is no off-chip SAW filter. In the proposed design, the TX front-end has three quadrature mixers, namely, the two low-frequency (LF) IQ mixers and the high-frequency (HF) IQ mixer, which convert the zero-IF-like ABB signal into dual RF bands. There are two cases (1) only one of the LF mixers is turned on, and the HF mixer is just bypassed, then the ABB signal is directly quadrature converted to 400 MHz RF signal by mixing with f_{LO_D} and (2) the two LF mixers generate IQ IF signals by using f_{LO_D} as their LO input, and these signals quadrature mixes with the IQ signals of f_{LO} to generate the 2.4 GHz single sideband RF signal using the HF mixer.

In this sliding-IF configuration, the IQ LO signals of the HF mixer are generated using a passive RC poly-phase filter (PPF). The up-converted signals from the in-phase LF mixer in (1) or the HF mixer in (2) are fed to the power amplifier (PA) depending on the switch selection.

The proposed transceiver architecture supports both 400 MHz and 2.4 GHz WBAN bands with the reconfigurable sliding-IF and zero-IF architecture. Note that some reported multiband WBAN transceivers with conventional architectures usually deploy two or more PLLs or RF front-ends [7, 9] for multiband operations. As a contrast, the proposed design greatly saves hardware and consequently lowers the cost.

4.4.1.2   Frequency Plan

For the architecture presented above, the frequency plan is one of the key issues that affect the reconfigurable transceiver performance. We mainly focus on the frequency plan for the 400 MHz and 2.4 GHz bands. Though the presented WBAN hub transceiver does not cover the 900 MHz band, this band is also considered for frequency interference and future design expansibility.

As shown in Fig. 4.18, the center frequency of ABB signal f_{ABB} is zero. When the proposed transceiver is configured to the sliding-IF mode for the 2.4 GHz band operation,

$$f_{LO} = \frac{f_{RF}}{1 \pm 1/2^n} \tag{4.5}$$

$$f_{IM} = \left(1 \mu 1/2^n\right) f_{LO} \tag{4.6}$$

The denominator in (4.5) is $(1+1/2^n)$ and $(1-1/2^n)$ for high-LO and low-LO configuration, respectively, and the opposite in (4.6). According to (4.5), there are two design freedoms in the frequency plan. One is to choose high-LO ($f_{LO}>f_{RF}$) or low-LO ($f_{LO}<f_{RF}$) conversion for the HF mixer, and the other is to set different values for n so that the divide-by-2^n divider can generate different LF mixer LO frequencies.

When the transceiver is configured to the zero-IF mode for the 400 MHz band operation,

$$f_{LO} = 2^n f_{RF} \tag{4.7}$$

In (4.7), if n simply increases by 1, the architecture can expand to support 900 MHz band without much changing in f_{LO}.

Given the operation frequency range in different modes, the required LO frequency tuning range for each band can be calculated using (4.5) and (4.7).

Three possible frequency plan schemes calculated from (4.5) and (4.7) are summarized in Table 4.4. 900 MHz band frequency plan is also listed for possible design expansibility. All the three schemes only require the VCO tuning range to be about 20 % as an advantage of the proposed reconfigurable sliding-IF architecture.

Table 4.4 Possible schemes of frequency planning

f_{RF} (MHz)		Scheme I	Scheme II	Scheme III
2,360–2,483.5	HB mixer type	Low-LO	Low-LO	High-LO
	$1/2^n$	1/2	1/4	1/4
	f_{LO} (MHz)	1,573–1,656	1,888–1,988	3,146–3,312
	f_{IM} (MHz)	786–828	1,416–1,491	3,933–4,140
402–450	$1/2^n$	1/4	1/4	1/8
	f_{LO} (MHz)	1,608–1,800	1,608–1,800	3,216–3,600
863–958	$1/2^n$	1/2	1/2	1/4
	f_{LO} (MHz)	1,726–1,916	1,726–1,916	3,452–3,832
All 3 bands	$1/2^n$	1/2, 1/4	1/2, 1/4	1/4, 1/8
	f_{LO} (MHz)	1,573–1,916	1,608–1,988	3,146–3,832
	Tuning range	19.8 %	21.1 %	19.8 %

When choosing the frequency plan, the IM frequency, the power consumption
related to LO frequency, and the complexity of the programmable frequency divider
should all be taken into consideration. Though the very high IM frequency in
scheme III makes the IM filtering more easily, the doubled frequency causes the
PLL and the LO distribution circuits to consume about twice of power. On the other
hand, schemes I and II use the low-LO configuration for the HF mixer and require a
much lower LO frequency and thus much lower power consumption compared to
the high-LO scheme III. However, the IM signal of scheme I is located around
800 MHz, which is too close to the 900 MHz WBAN band. Scheme II was chosen
in the proposed transceiver finally for its low power consumption and the acceptable
IM frequency. The IM signal in scheme II actually ranges from 1,416 to 1,491 MHz
(allocated to satellites application) and is far from the 400 MHz, 900 MHz, and the
2.4 GHz possible WBAN signal bands so that sufficient IM suppression can be
achieved using just the LC resonances in the LNA (RX) and the up-mixer (TX).

Figure 4.19 visualizes the frequency conversion mechanisms and the required
LO frequency range of the selected frequency plan. With the proposed architecture
and the frequency planning, the LO only needs an output range of 1,608–1,988 MHz,
which can significantly alleviate the design requirements on the LO circuit as compared to the over designed SDR architecture.

4.4.2   Circuits Design

4.4.2.1   **Wideband RF Front-End**

Active Shunt Feedback LNA with Multiple G_m Enhancement

A wideband LNA is shown in Fig. 4.20 together with a PA and their shared matching
balun.

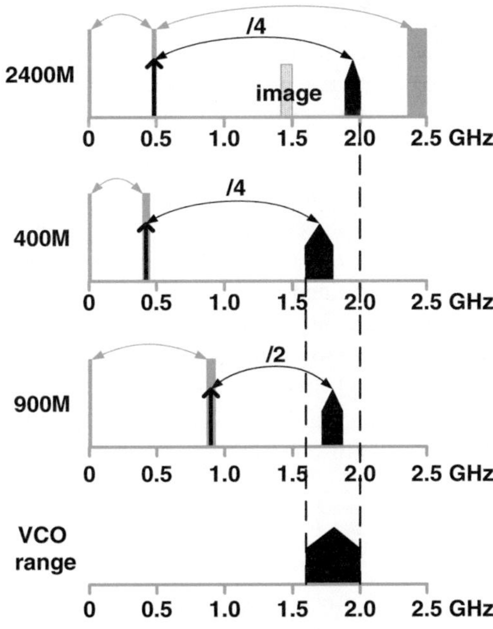

Fig. 4.19 Multiband frequency conversion mechanisms and needed VCO tunning range

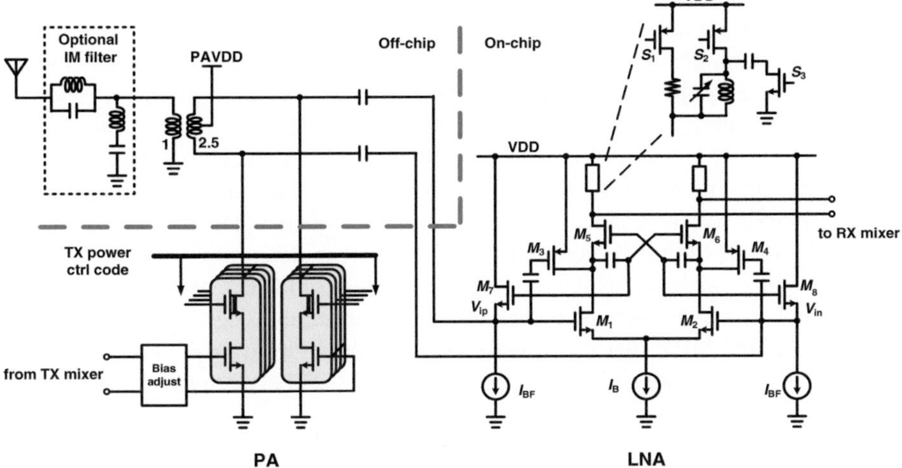

Fig. 4.20 wideband RF front-end and off-chip matching circuits

In the LNA, the NMOS input pair M_1/M_2 provides the amplifier's transconductance (G_m). The PMOS M_3/M_4 are introduced as a parallel input pair to enhance the overall G_m. Particularly, M_3 and M_4 conduct most part of the tail current I_B, so large load resistors can be used to boost the LNA gain without imposing any extra DC voltage headroom so that the receiver can use a low supply voltage to maintain the low power consumption.

The LNA uses the active shunt feedback for wideband input matching with the cascode transistors M_5/M_6 and source follower transistors M_7/M_8 forming the active feedback path and giving a wideband resistance characteristic:

$$Z_{in} = \frac{2}{g_{m7,8}\left(1 + G_{m,in}Z_C\right)} \tag{4.8}$$

where $g_{m7,8}$ stands for transconductance of M_7/M_8, $G_{m,in}$ is the total G_m of the input transistors M_1/M_2 and M_3/M_4, and Z_C is the impedance at the cascode node and is mainly determined by the node parasitic capacitance and cascode G_m. To overcome the large parasitic capacitance contributed by all the transistors, M_5 and M_6 connected in the cross-coupled structure are used to enhance the cascode G_m so as to flatten the high-frequency input impedance. Also, the enhanced G_m helps to avoid high-frequency noise performance declining due to the cascode node capacitance. The overall noise factor (F_n) is given by:

$$F_n = 1 + \frac{\gamma}{\alpha}\left(\frac{1}{1 + G_{m,in}/2g_{m5,6}} + \frac{1}{R_S G_{m,in}}\right) + \frac{1}{R_S R_L G_{m,in}^2} \tag{4.9}$$

where γ is the excess channel thermal noise coefficient, and α, approximately equal to 1, is the ratio between the transconductance and the zero-bias drain conductance of the input transistor. R_S and R_L stand for the source and load resistance, respectively. Equations 4.8 and 4.9 show that the proposed LNA architecture provides a flat input matching impedance and an optimized NF simultaneously over a wide frequency range and avoids the trade-off between the impedance matching and NF performance usually seen in the common gate LNA [20].

The LNA load is designed to switch between a resistor and an LC tank as shown in Figure 4.20. The resistor load provides a wideband gain in 400 MHz operation mode, while the LC resonance enhances the high frequency gain and filters out the IM signal in the sliding-IF configuration. The IRR is determined by the Q-factor which is mainly impacted by the turning on resistance of PMOS switch S_2. However, large switch size may introduce parasitic capacitance, and degrade the gain when working in 400 MHz. An additional capacitor through an NMOS switch S_3 to ground has been introduced to provide a good trade-off between the 400 MHz and the 2.4 GHz selections.

Class AB/B/C Reconfigurable PA

As shown in Fig. 4.20, the PA uses a pseudo-differential common-source cascode configuration to maximize the available output swing headroom at the low supply. The 1.8-V normal-gate transistors are used for the input transconductance stage for both high gain and high speed, while the 3.3-V thick-gate devices are used as the cascode transistors for the reliability consideration since the inductance loads raise the transient peak output voltage up to about twice of the supply voltage PAVDD.

The cascode PA is formed by a series of parallel transistors. Its output power is programmable from −10 to +3 dBm depending on the number of branches switched on by a digital code. To avoid the PA efficiency degradation related to nonideal switches inserted to the PA branches, all the programmable branches are controlled by the cascode transistors. The cascode devices' gates are biased to ground or VDD for turning off/on the branches, respectively. Choosing VDD as the cascode gate voltage helps to maximize the V_{DS} of the input transconductance transistors and therefore to maintain the PA linearity. The side effect of little headroom for the PA output node voltage has been minimized through careful design, and the output 1 dB compression degradation associated with this choice can be neglected. The input signal swing and the DC biased voltage of the input transistor are adjustable to configure the PA working conditions under different situations. In this design, the PA conduction angle can be adjusted from about 120° to 320°. When the transceiver is used for IEEE 802.15.6 NB π/2-DBPSK or π/4-DQPSK, the PA works as a class AB one, to ensure the required linearity. When it is used for the constant-envelope modulation (OQPSK for ZigBee and MSK for the wireless endoscope capsule system), class B or C operation is more preferred for good PA efficiency.

Matching Circuits Shared by RX/TX

The differential input of the LNA and the output of the PA are converted to a single-ended 50 Ω antenna through a wideband balun. The on-chip wideband balun covering frequency as low as 400 MHz needs a large area and its 400 MHz band insertion loss is large due to the low Q-factor in low frequency limited by the available CMOS process. As a result, an off-chip balun has been adopted in this design. To make the PA and the LNA share the same RF port, the powered-off PA's output impedance and the disabled LNA's input impedance are designed large enough to be negligible.

For the LNA, a high balun-turns ratio, which means the 50 Ω antenna impedance is transformed to a high terminal impedance, is preferred for low-noise performance since it favors voltage amplification [21]. However, the LNA input impedance will decline at high frequency due to input node parasitic capacitance C_{ip}. In this design, including the PA output node capacitance (the PA is powered off in RX mode), C_{ip} is about 200 fF which results in a reactance of about 350 Ω at 2.4 GHz. The reasonable input impedance mainly determined by $g_{m7,8}$ in (4.4) should be no more than 350 Ω to flatten the input reflection in all the desired bands. On the other hand, the PA requires optimum load impedance to trade-off between efficiency and output power as given by:

$$R_{OPT} = \frac{2\left(V_{DD} - V_{knee}\right)^2}{P_{out}} \tag{4.10}$$

where $(V_{DD} - V_{knee})$ means the available PA output amplitude and is about 0.8 V in this design. P_{out} is the desired output power and is chosen as +6 dBm for +3 dBm

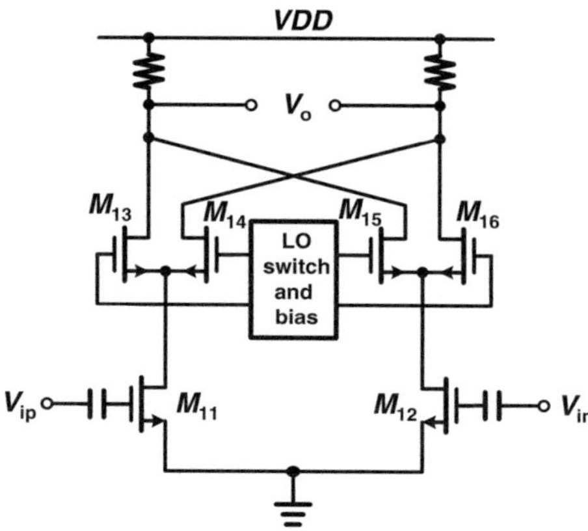

Fig. 4.21 Reconfigurable HF amp-mix

maximum output and about 3 dB loss in balun and others. The optimum load is then 320 Ω. Finally, a 1:2.5 balun is chosen to satisfy both RX and TX requirements.

An optional external second-order band-stop LC filter can be inserted between the antenna and the balun. This filter can help to further suppress IM signal in 1.4~1.5 GHz when the transceiver works in the sliding-IF mode. It provides an additional IRR improvement of 20 dB. However, without this off-chip filter, the on-chip LC resonant loads of the LNA in RX and the HF mixer in TX can still offer sufficient IRR for basic WBAN applications.

4.4.2.2   Reconfigurable RX Mixer

Figure 4.21 shows the RX HF amp-mix circuits. It acts as a Gilbert mixer with a high-frequency LO input, and serves as an amplifier while the LO input is just a DC signal. In the mixer mode, NMOS $M_{13}-M_{16}$ are biased to act as the active switches driven by LO. While in the amplifier mode, NMOS M_{14} and M_{15} are turned off, and M_{13} and M_{16} are biased to form a pseudo-differential cascode amplifier with M_{11} and M_{12}, in which M_{11}/M_{12} act as the common-source input stage and M_{13}/M_{16} act as the cascode transistors. When operated in the mixer mode, to suppress the IM the LNA's resistor load is switched to an LC tank to filter out the noise and interference signal in the image frequency band as discussed above.

Figure 4.22 illustrates one path of the RX LF quadrature mixer. The PMOS input and switch transistors are used for good flick noise performance. To get a high output voltage swing, the NMOS active load is chosen. The load G_m is limited by cutting down the bias current for differential noise reduction. A common mode (CM) feed-back circuit is designed to collect the redundant current and to stabilize the output CM voltage.

When receiving 400 MHz signal, the additional HF amp-mix results in some extra power consumption and die area compared to the classic direct conversion zero-IF receiver, which is the penalty of the proposed architecture. Nevertheless, this extra

Fig. 4.22 One path of RX
LF quadrature mixer with
high-swing low-noise load

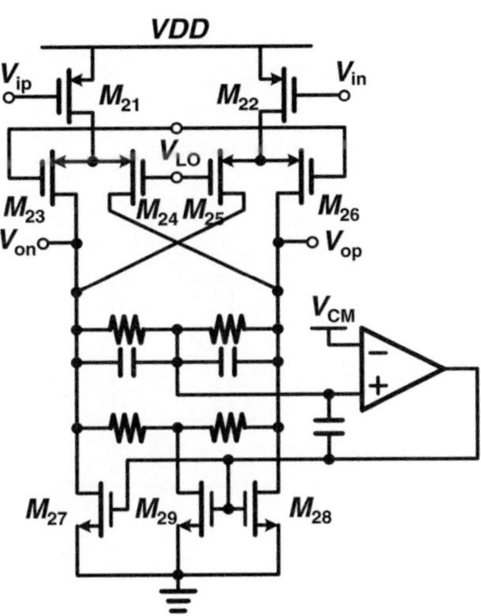

stage provides about 10 dB additional gain, which helps to suppress the noise contribution of the LF quadrature mixer. Actually, with the proposed architecture, the
extra gain contributed by the HF amp-mix shifts the RX flick noise corner frequency
from about 120 kHz to below 25 kHz, which benefits the subsequent baseband
demodulation.

4.4.2.3   Reconfigurable TX Mixer

Figure 4.23 shows the simplified TX up-mixer structure. A second-order PPF is
used to generate the IQ LO signals for the HF mixer. This PPF exhibits approximately 35 dB image rejection in 1,880–2,000 MHz band with 15 % resistance variation and 5 % capacitance variation [22]. The PPF order and RC values are chosen
with the trade-off between the IRR and the LO driver power consumption.
An inductor is used to resonate with the PPF equivalent capacitor so as to deliver
large amplitude IQ LO signals to the HF mixer. In addition, the HF mixer uses an
LC tank load to filter out 1.4~1.5 GHz IM signal.

4.4.2.4   Frequency Synthesizer

A fully integrated synthesizer is designed using a third-order Σ–Δ fractional-N PLL
as illustrated in Fig. 4.18. A 1.5~2.1 GHz LC tank VCO fully covers the required
21 % LO frequency range (1.608–1.988 GHz) in any process, voltage, and temperature
corners.

A large KVCO may degrade the phase noise performance through AM-to-PM
noise conversion [21]. To alleviate this issue, the VCO frequency is coarsely controlled
by an 8-bit digitally switched capacitor bank to avoid a large KVCO throughout the

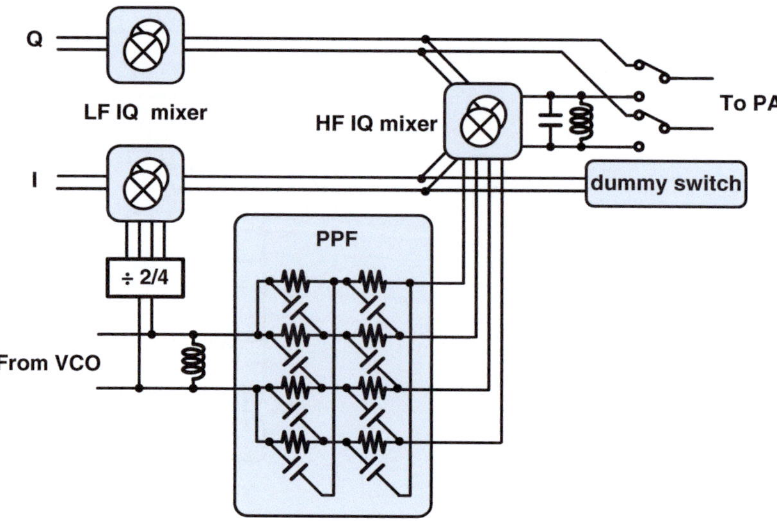

Fig. 4.23 Simplified TX up-converter with PPF IQ LO generator

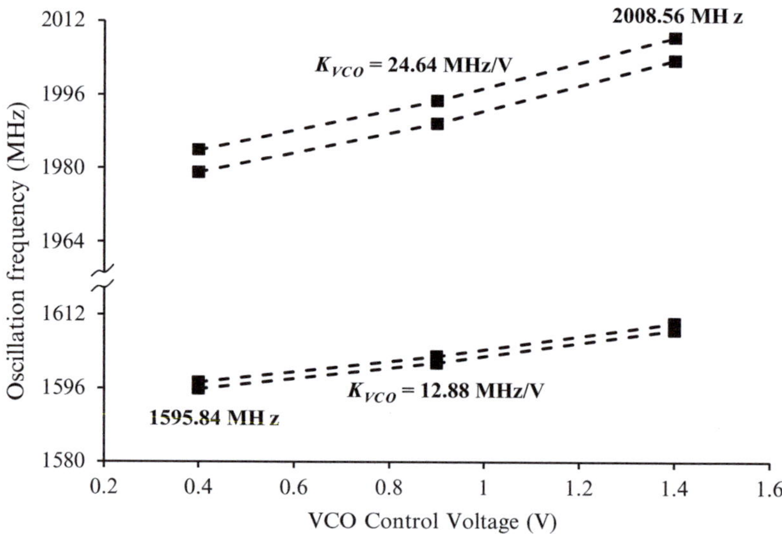

Fig. 4.24 Measured KVCO variation with switched-capacitor bank setting

entire tuning range. The capacitor bank setting is determined using a fast frequency-lock algorithm before the phase-lock operation. Note that KVCO varies with the capacitor bank setting as shown in Fig. 4.24 (only show the voltage control curves with the lowest and the highest switched capacitor). The charge pump (CP) current is designed to change with KVCO adaptively to maintain the PLL loop bandwidth around 150 kHz.

4.4.2.5   RX and TX IF

The RX ABB includes a 150 kHz to 3 MHz bandwidth reconfigurable low-pass filter (LPF), a three stages 0–60 dB PGA and an 8-bit 12 Msps successive approximation ADC in both I and Q paths, respectively. A look-up-table (LUT) free DC offset calibration method is introduced to remove the PGA-gain-correlated offset residue [23].

The TX ABB includes an 8-bit 24 Msps current-steering DAC and a bandwidth reconfigurable LPF (identical to that used in RX) in both I and Q paths, respectively. The high DAC sample rate moves the DAC image components and the clock leakage to high frequencies, so that the integrated ABB filter can easily suppress those unwanted frequency components for excellent alternate channel power rejection (ACPR).

The bandwidth reconfigurable filters in both RX and TX are a third-order active-RC filter with programmable capacitors. The core opamp of the filter is designed using an adaptive Miller compensation structure, which makes the stability of the amplifier not affected by the bandwidth changing [24]. An on-chip RC calibration circuits is shared by both RX and TX.

4.4.3   Implementation Results

The transceiver is designed and fabricated in 0.18 μm CMOS process. Figure 4.25 shows its die photograph. The chip size is 4×4 mm^2, of which only 6.1 mm^2 is used by the RF, analog and PMU. The transceiver achieves a high level of integration, and the required external components are just a 1:2.5 RF balun, a 24 MHz crystal, a 24 kΩ resistor for current bias generation, three 1 μF capacitors for on-chip LDO regulators, and an optional external RF LC bandstop filter before the antenna to suppress the IM signal when configured in sliding-IF architecture (no SAW filter is needed).

Figure 4.26 shows the measured phase noise of the buffered out PLL divided-by-4 signal. The phase noise at 1 MHz offset of the carrier frequency is −121.5 dBc/Hz, which outperforms those 400 MHz single band designs for WBAN applications [8]. Assuming the divided-by-4 signal has 12 dB better phase noise performance, the original PLL phase noise in 2 GHz is then about −109.5 dBc/Hz at 1 MHz offset, which is comparable to other 2.4 GHz transceivers [9, 11, 12].

Figure 4.27 shows the NF of the receiver from the input port of the RF balun to the analog test buffer that connects to the last stage of ABB. The measurement was performed at the maximum RX gain setting. Thanks to the high voltage gain of the 1:2.5 balun and the LNA, the total RX chain NF is below 4.4 dB for the 2.4 GHz band, and below 3.9 dB for the 400 MHz band.

When the receiver works at the 2.4 GHz sliding-IF mode with the maximum RX gain, the total RX chain gain is 98 dB for the 2.4 GHz desired signal, whereas only 64 dB for the 1.5 GHz image signal with the filtering effect of the LNA load resonator, which indicates the RX sliding-IF IRR is about 34 dB.

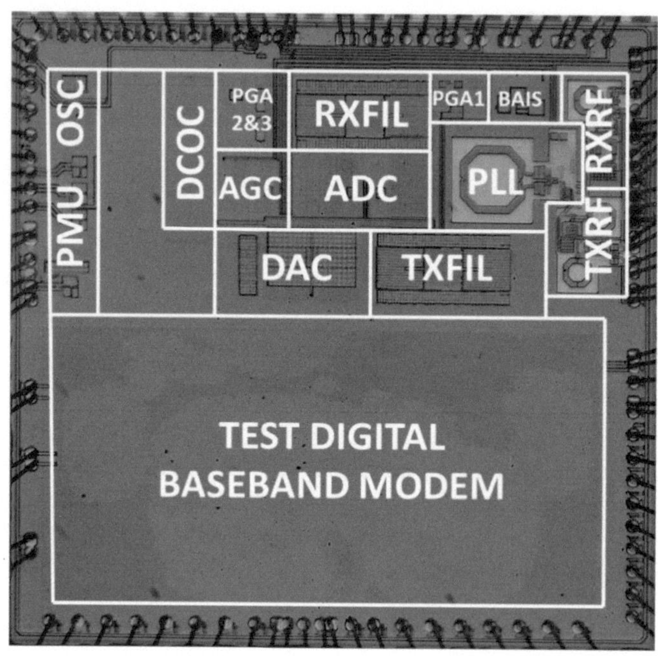

Fig. 4.25 Micrograph of 2.4 GHz PBS transceiver

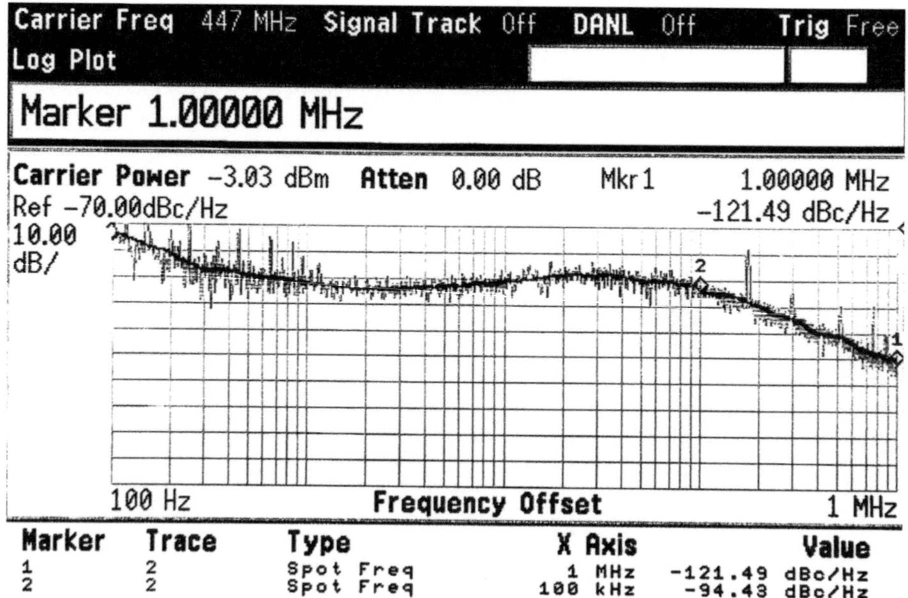

Fig. 4.26 Measured phase noise of PLL divided-by-4 output

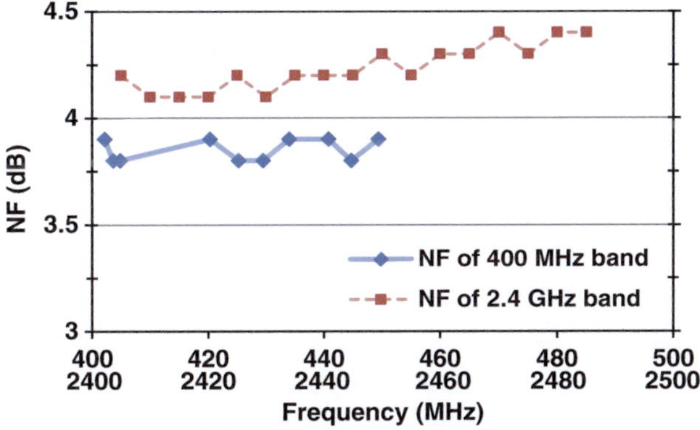

Fig. 4.27 Measured noise figure of whole receiver at 400 MHz and 2.4 GHz bands

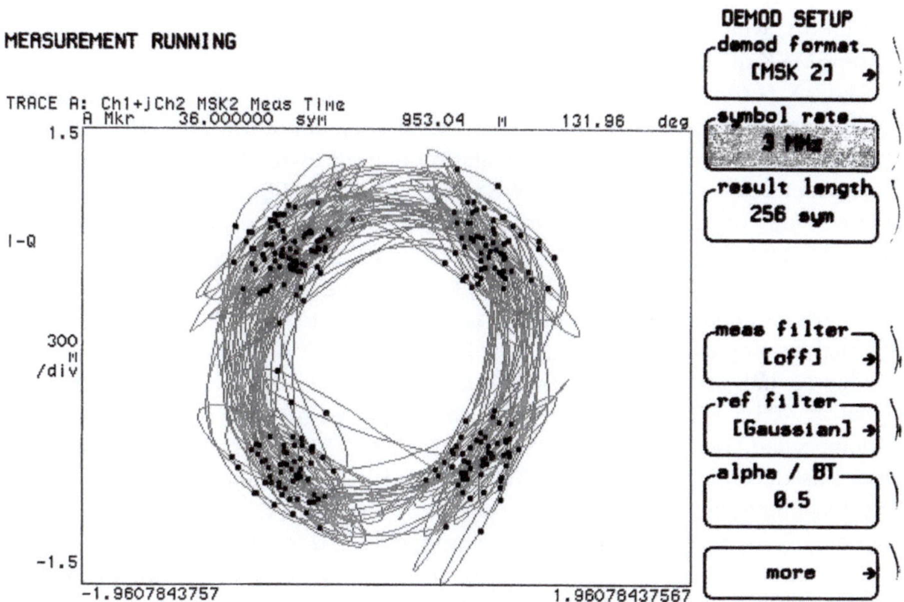

Fig. 4.28 Measured RX ABB signal constellation diagram with RF input at −90 dBm 3 Mbps
MSK

Figure 4.28 shows the measured ABB signal constellation diagram at the highest
data rate of 3 Mbps for the wireless endoscope capsule application. In the measurement, a vector signal generator is used to output a 417 MHz 3 Mbps MSK signal
at −90 dBm power level to the receiver input port, and the analog LPF bandwidth
is configured to 3 MHz. The measured ABB error vector magnitude (EVM) is
23 %, which means the demodulator can have an input signal-to-noise ratio (SNR)

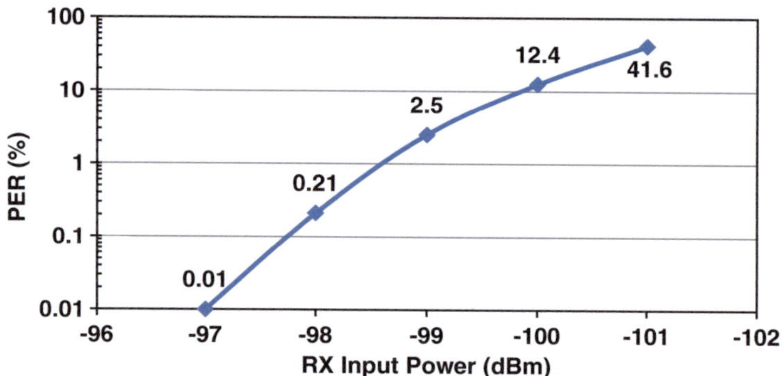

Fig. 4.29 Measured PER versus RX input power of 2,425 MHz 250 kbps ZigBee 20 octets PSDU packet

of 12.8 dB, which is adequate for demodulation. The measured RX sensitivity of 3 Mbps MSK at 10^{-3} BER is −89 dBm.

The RX performance for 2.4 GHz ZigBee compliant has been tested under the conditions as specified in the receiver sensitivity definition of IEEE 802.15.4 standards [4]. A NI virtual instrumentation is used to send a stream of packets. The packet size is set with the PHY Service Data Unit (PSDU) length equal to 20 octets. A total of 32,768 packets are sent and the number of packets not detected or failed in demodulation are counted to calculate the packets error rate (PER). Figure 4.29 shows the measured PER verses RX input power level, and the 1 % PER sensitivity is about −99 dBm, which is comparable to the −94 to −101 dBm as reported for single band ZigBee transceivers [10–12].

Figures 4.30 and 4.31 show the TX output spectrum of 187.5 kbp π/4-DQPSK signal at 403.5 MHz and −3.7 dBm output power in class-AB mode and the 2 Mchip/s half sine sharped O-QPSK signal at 2,425 MHz and +1.6 dBm in class-C mode, as defined by the IEEE 802.15.6 and ZigBee standards, respectively. The reconfigurable transmitter has exhibited quite good linearity performance in both modes and meets the specified spectrum masks, respectively.

Figure 4.32 is the constellation diagram of the transmitted ZigBee signal at 2.425 GHz. The measured EVM of 1,000 symbols is 8 %, which satisfies the standard (35 %) quite well. Further simulation has indicated that the EVM can be improved with more symmetrical layout.

Figure 4.33 shows the measured PA efficiency when biased in the different modes for 400 MHz and 2.4 GHz operation, respectively. The maximum output power is +4.7 dBm and +3.1 dBm with the PAE 40 % and 31 % at 400 MHz and 2.4 GHz, respectively. Note that the PA was optimized only for large output levels, the PAE drops when reducing the PA gain setting, as shown in Fig. 4.33.

Figure 4.34 shows the measured wide-range spectrum when transmitting a 2.416 GHz signal at the +3 dBm level. The measured spectrum shows that the LO leakage is −43.8 dBc, and the TX sliding-IF IRR is 47.1 dBc.

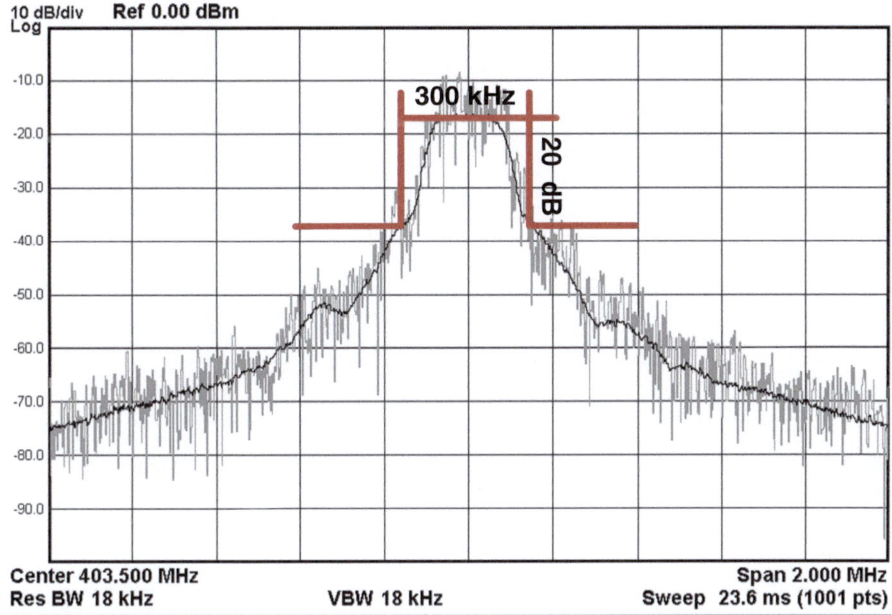

Fig. 4.30 Measured TX spectrum of 187.5 kbps π/4-DQPSK signal at 403.5 MHz

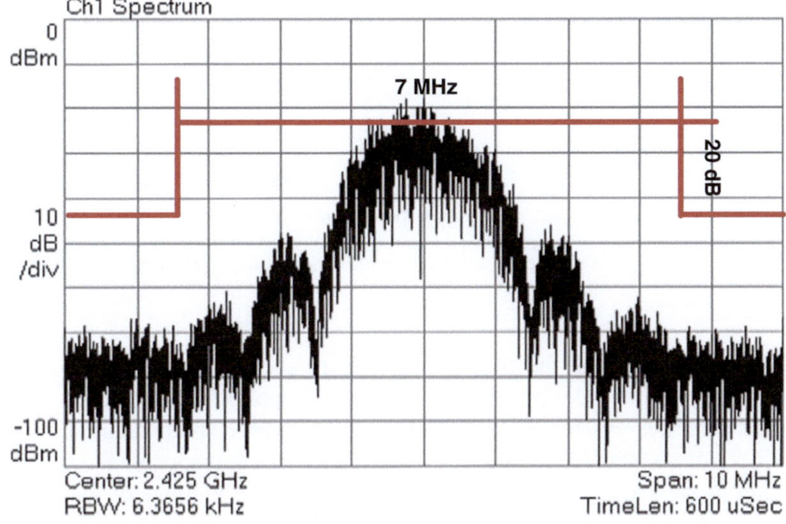

Fig. 4.31 Measured TX spectrum of 2 Mchip/s O-QPSK (ZigBee) signal at 2,425 MHz

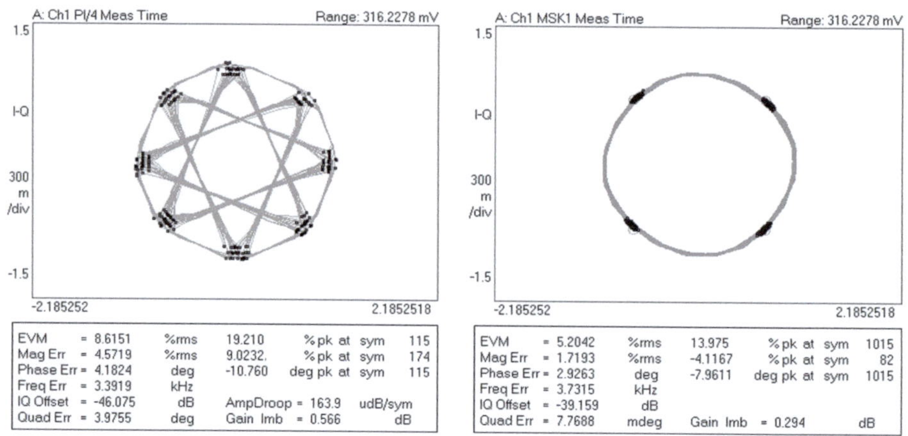

Fig. 4.32 Measured transmitter constellation diagram at 2.425 GHz. (**a**) 600 kbps π/4-DQPSK signal, (**b**) ZigBee signal

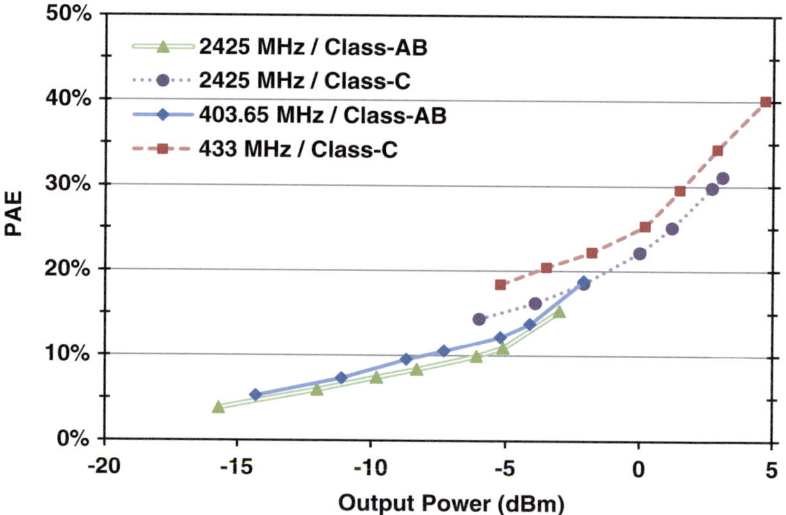

Fig. 4.33 Measured TX PA efficiency of different bias condition at 400 MHz and 2.4 GHz bands

Table 4.5 summarizes the transceiver performance and gives the comparison between this dual-band design and the previously reported SDR designs as well as the single band designs for WBAN/ZigBee in literature. The presented dual-band transceiver covers 400 MHz and 2.4 GHz bands simultaneously. If we limit the discussion to the scope of WBAN/ZigBee applications which needs discontinuous and narrow band covering, the presented transceiver has less complicated circuit structure and consumes less power than the SDR transceivers [13, 25] when used

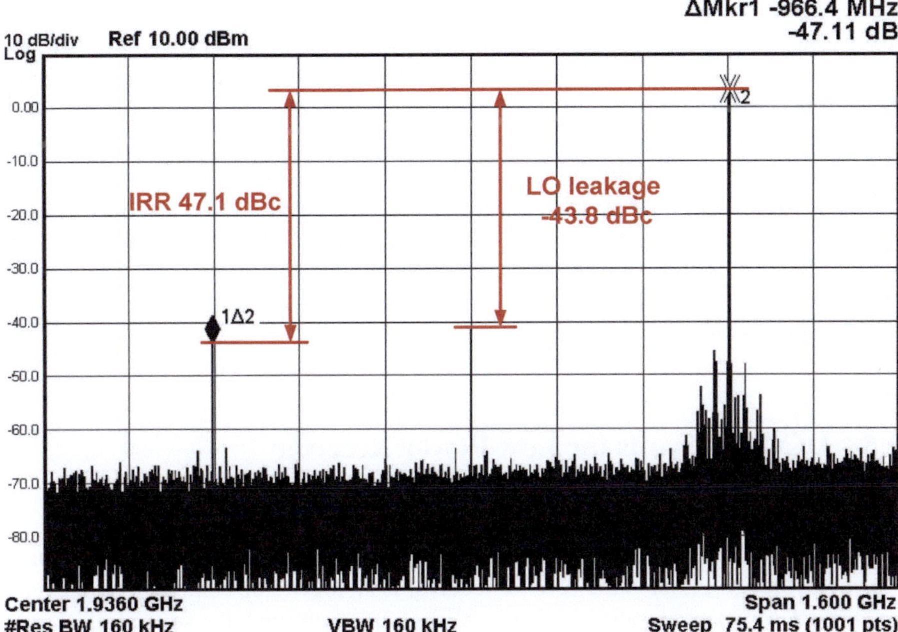

Fig. 4.34 Measured TX wideband spectrum when transmit at 2.416 GHz single frequency signal

Table 4.5 PBS transceiver performance summary

Technology	180 nm CMOS	
Frequency (GHz)	0.36–0.51	2.36–2.5
Supply voltage (V)	1.55	
RX NF (dB)	3.9	4.4
RX in-band IIP3 (dBm)	−29.4	−26.6
ABB bandwidth (MHz)	0.15–3	
RX power (mW)	15.8	16.6
TX Max P_{out} (dBm)	+4.7	+3.1
TX power (mW) @ Max P_{out}	13.2	18.0
VCO range	21 %	
Phase noise @ 1 MHz (dBc/Hz)	−121.5	−109.5[4]
Area (mm^2)	6.1	

for these specific applications. The proposed reconfigurable sliding-IF architecture reduces the required VCO tuning range significantly, and thus dramatically alleviates the design difficulties and saves power consumption. Compared to the previously reported single band counterparts [7–12], this new design has achieved comparable or even better performance in terms of noise, RX sensitivity, phase noise, power consumption, and even die area while covering both 400 MHz and 2.4 GHz frequency bands.

In summary, a low-power PBS transceiver for dual-band WBAN hubs is discussed in this section. A novel reconfigurable sliding-IF transceiver architecture has been proposed which relaxes the frequency synthesizer tuning range to only 21 % while supporting WBAN hubs that cover both the 400 MHz and 2.4 GHz frequency bands.

Measurement results on the designed and fabricated dual-band transceiver in 0.18 μm shows that it has comparable or even better performance in terms of noise, RX sensitivity, phase noise, power consumption, and even die area compared to the single band transceivers in literature, while providing the unique frequency band coverage of both the 400 MHz and 2.4 GHz, which will greatly facilitates the WBAN hubs with superb compatibility and flexibility.

4.5   DCOC Circuits for Low Power Receiver

The zero-IF architecture is becoming a superior one among wireless transceiver architectures for its advantages in image rejection and low power IF circuits. However, the DC offset in the zero-IF receiver is an inevitable challenge. Offset can be caused by many modules of a receiver and amplified by several IF PGA. Sometimes, it can easily saturate the tail stage analog circuits and ADC in the IF circuits. To cancel the effect of the offset, many circuits have been developed. All in all, the conventional DC offset cancellation (DCOC) circuits can be classified into two sorts, the analog circuit and the mixed-signal one.

The commonly used analog DCOC technique is the AC coupling and analog feedback [26–28]. These circuits are usually adopted in low-IF receivers. The DC operation voltages of AC coupled modules are independent of each other, which is the simplest way to maintain the DC bias stable. Analog feedback circuits usually get the output offset voltage with an integrator and subtract it from the input voltage. However, AC coupling and analog feedback circuits eliminate not only the DC offset but also some low-frequency signal. Those circuits can be viewed as high-pass filter in frequency domain and the equivalent cutoff frequency are supposed to be low enough to avoid distortion of the received signal. So, large resistors and capacitors are required to achieve a low cutoff frequency, which leads to huge die area. Also, a low cutoff frequency leads to a long setup time. Just because of the referred problems, analog DCOC techniques can hardly be used in zero-IF receivers.

The conventional mixed-signal DCOC circuits detect the output DC offset and trim the IF circuits with DAC [29, 30]. Typically, a receiver requires an RF gain of 30 dB and an IF gain of 60 dB or even larger to keep the dynamic range. A large LUT is required to store all the DCOC trim bits since the output DC offset is relative to the RF and IF gains of the receiver.

In this section, a novel mixed signal DCOC circuits independent of IF gain for zero-IF receiver applications will be discussed. By avnalyzing the offset model and arranging the gain of every IF PGA, the residue output offset voltage can be well controlled. The new DCOC circuit calibrates the DC offset only at maximum gain and saves 98 % memory area compared to a conventional circuit, which calibrates DC offsets at all IF gains.

Fig. 4.35 (a) Input referred offset model, (b) output referred offset model

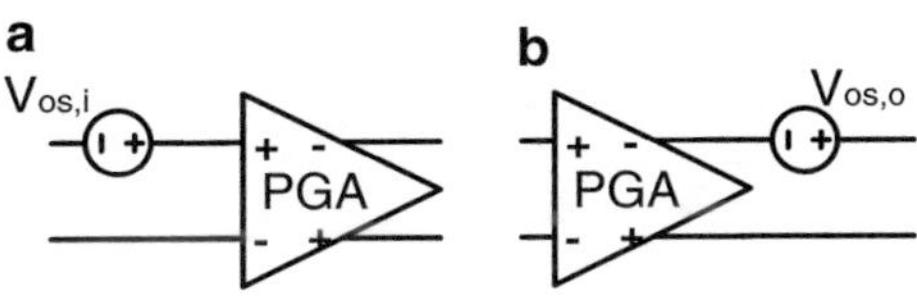

Fig. 4.36 A new DC offset model

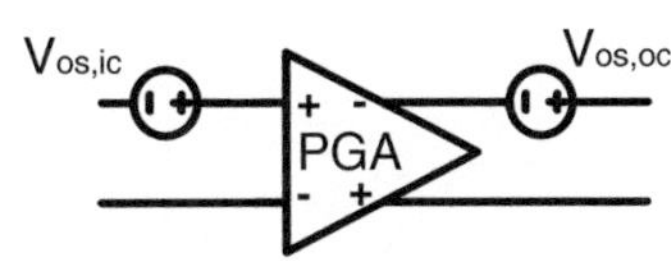

4.5.1   Offset Models and Calibration Method

4.5.1.1   DC Offset Models

Traditionally, the DC offset is modeled as a DC voltage source shown in Fig. 4.35. A practical amplifier can be viewed as an ideal PGA and an equivalent offset source in the input or the output [31].

The input referred offset voltage $V_{os,i}$ and the output referred offset voltage $V_{os,o}$ are all correlated to the gain of PGA. A is the gain of the amplifier, then:

$$V_{os,i} = AV_{os,o} \tag{4.11}$$

A new model is reported in [32]. As is shown in Fig. 4.36, the new model divided the offset voltage into two parts. $V_{os,ic}$ is the input part and $V_{os,oc}$ is the output part. They are constant at all PGA gains. It is proved that the new model can be applied to most of amplifier structures.

The total DC offset can be expressed as:

$$V_{os} = AV_{os,ic} + V_{os,oc} \tag{4.12}$$

With the new model, the DC offset of a zero-IF receiver can be given in Fig. 4.37a. $V_{oc,m}$ is the output offset of down mixer. $V_{ic,p1}$ and $V_{oc,p1}$ are the input and output part of PGA1 offset. $V_{oc,f}$ is the output offset of IF filter. $V_{ic,p2}$ and $V_{oc,p2}$ are the input and output part of PGA2 offset. $V_{ic,p3}$ and $V_{oc,p3}$ are the input and output part of PGA3 offset.

$V_{oc,m}$ and $V_{ic,p1}$ can be obviously replaced by one voltage source V_{os0}. Similarly, $V_{oc,p1}$, $V_{oc,f}$, and $V_{ic,p2}$ are replaced by V_{os1}. $V_{oc,p2}$ and $V_{ic,p3}$ are replaced by V_{os2}. $V_{oc,p3}$ are rewritten as V_{os3}. Then, a simplified DC offset model independent of PGA gain is given in Fig. 4.37b.

Usually, V_{os0}, V_{os1}, V_{os2}, and V_{os3} vary from 0 to 20 mV. Total output DC offset is as follow:

$$V_{os} = A_1 A_2 A_3 V_{os0} + A_2 A_3 V_{os1} + A_3 V_{os2} + V_{os3} \tag{4.13}$$

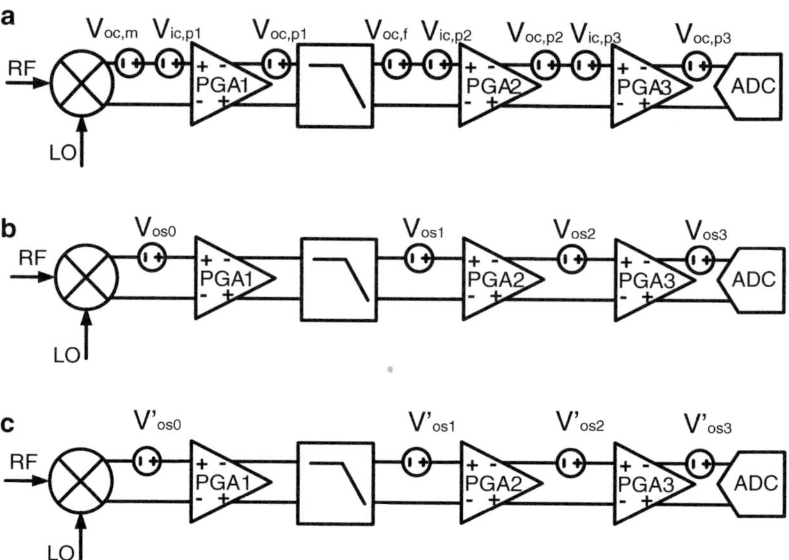

Fig. 4.37 (**a**) DC offset model of zero-IF receiver, (**b**) simplified DC offset model, (**c**) residue DC offset

where, A_1, A_2, and A_3 are the gains of PGA1, PGA2, and PGA3 individually. They are 0–20 dB typically. Although V_{os0}, V_{os1}, V_{os2}, and V_{os3} are independent of A_1, A_2, and A_3, the total output offset is correlated to the gains. Next, we present a novel method that keeps the total output residue offset voltage approximately constant when the IF gain changes.

4.5.1.2   A Novel DC Offset Calibration Method

The novel DCOC method consists of two major steps:

1. Calibrate once at maximum IF gain
2. Adjust the IF gain in the certain sequence shown in Fig. 4.38

It is explained in detail as follows.

First, A_1, A_2, and A_3 are set to maximum. Simple analog or mixed signal methods can be used to calibrate every part of offset. V_{os0}, V_{os1}, V_{os2}, and V_{os3} are minimized to quite small (typically below 5 mV). Every part of the residue offset is shown in Fig. 4.37c and the total residue output DC offset voltage is written as:

$$V'_{os} = A_1 A_2 A_3 V'_{os0} + A_2 A_3 V'_{os1} + A_3 V'_{os2} + V'_{os3} \tag{4.14}$$

And then:

$$A_1 A_2 A_3 V'_{os0} + A_2 A_3 V'_{os1} + A_3 V'_{os2} = V'_{os} - V'_{os3} \tag{4.15}$$

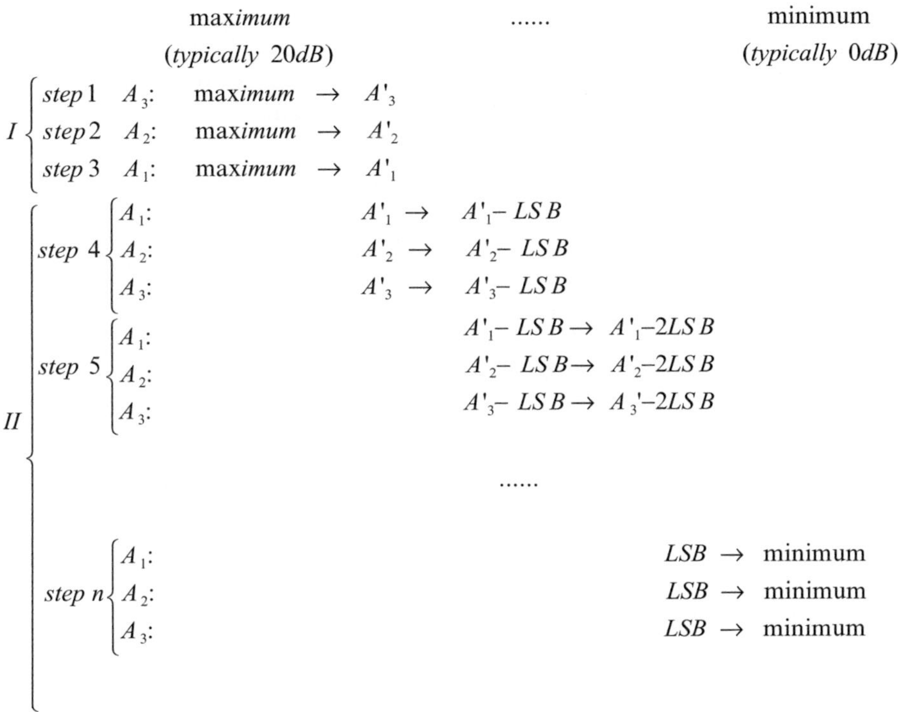

Fig. 4.38   Proposed IF gain arrangement

Second, the IF PGAs' gains are arranged in a novel way. When the automatic gain control (AGC) module of a receiver detects a very small signal, A_1, A_2, and A_3 are set to maximum and the residue offset has been calibrated. If AGC module detects a large signal, A_1, A_2, and A_3 will be decreased in a certain sequence as is shown in Fig. 4.38. A'_1, A'_2, and A'_3 are the intermediate gains of PGA1, PGA2, and PGA3. A_3, A_2, and A_1 are decreased to A'_3, A'_2, and A'_1 individually in part I. Then, A'_1, A'_2, and A'_3 are sequentially decreased to 0 dB in part II. The residue offsets of every step are analyzed as below:

$$V_{step1} = A_1 A_2 A'_3 V'_{os0} + A_2 A'_3 V'_{os1} + A'_3 V'_{os2} + V'_{os3}$$

$$= \left(V'_{os} - V'_{os3} \right) \frac{A'_3}{A_3} + V'_{os3}$$

$$= \underbrace{\frac{A'_3}{A_3} V'_{os}}_{item1} + \underbrace{\left(1 - \frac{A'_3}{A_3} \right) V'_{os3}}_{item2} \tag{4.16}$$

A'_1, A'_2, and A'_3 are supposed to be small (typically below 10 dB). After step1, the total output residue offset is calculated as (4.16). Equation 4.15 is used to simplify (4.16). Since $|V'_{os}|$ is small and A'_3/A_3 is below 1, the absolute value of item1 is even smaller than $|V'_{os}|$ and can be ignored. Similarly, since $|V'_{os3}|$ is small and

$1-A'_3/A_3$ is below 1, the absolute value of item2 is smaller than $|V'_{os3}|$ and can be ignored too. So, $|V_{step1}|$ is quite small, which means the output residue offset is approximately constant when the gain of PGA3 is decreased from maximum to A'_3.

After step2, the total output residue offset is calculated as:

$$V_{step2} = A_1 A'_2 A'_3 V'_{os0} + A'_2 A'_3 V'_{os1} + A'_3 V'_{os2} + V'_{os3}$$

$$= \left(V'_{os} - V'_{os3}\right)\frac{A'_2 A'_3}{A_2 A_3} - \frac{A'_2}{A_2} A'_3 V'_{os2} + A'_3 V'_{os2} + V'_{os3}$$

$$= \underbrace{\frac{A'_2 A'_3}{A_2 A_3} V'_{os}}_{item1} + \underbrace{\left(1 - \frac{A'_2}{A_2}\right) A'_3 V'_{os2}}_{item2} + \underbrace{\left(1 - \frac{A'_2 A'_3}{A_2 A_3}\right) V'_{os3}}_{item3} \tag{4.17}$$

The item1 and item3 can be proved to be ignorable. As A'_3 is below 10 dB, item2 is typically one or two times of V'_{os2} and can be ignored. So, $|V_{step2}|$ is quite small, which means the output residue offset is approximately constant when the gain of PGA2 is decreased from maximum to A'_2.

After step3, the total output residue offset is as (4.18).

$$V_{step3} = A'_1 A'_2 A'_3 V'_{os0} + A'_2 A'_3 V'_{os1} + A'_3 V'_{os2} + V'_{os3}$$

$$= \underbrace{\frac{A'_1 A'_2 A'_3}{A_1 A_2 A_3} V'_{os}}_{item1} + \underbrace{\left(1 - \frac{A'_1}{A_1}\right) A'_2 A'_3 V'_{os1}}_{item2}$$

$$+ \underbrace{\left(1 - \frac{A'_1 A'_2}{A_1 A_2}\right) A'_3 V'_{os2}}_{item3} + \underbrace{\left(1 - \frac{A'_1 A'_2 A'_3}{A_1 A_2 A_3}\right) V'_{os3}}_{item4} \tag{4.18}$$

Similarly, the item1, item3, and item4 can be proved to be small. But, item2 may vary greatly with A'_3, A'_2, and A'_1. $|V'_{os1}|$, $|V'_{os2}|$, and $|V'_{os3}|$ can be easily reduced below 5 mV. By assuming V'_{os1}, V'_{os2}, and V'_{os3} of the same sign and A'_3, A'_2, and A'_1 of the same value, the maximum output residue offset is shown in Fig. 4.39.

Apparently, the theoretical maximum residue offset of step3 is positively correlated with the intermediate gain. Small A'_3, A'_2, and A'_1 can be adopted to reduce V_{step3}.

After step4, step5, and stepn, the total output residue offset V_{step4}, V_{step5}, and V_{stepn} are written as:

$$V_{step4} = V_{step3}\Big|_{A'_1 = A'_1 - LSB, A'_2 = A'_2 - LSB, A'_3 = A'_3 - LSB} \tag{4.19}$$

$$V_{step5} = V_{step3}\Big|_{A'_1 = A'_1 - 2LSB, A'_2 = A'_2 - 2LSB, A'_3 = A'_3 - 2LSB} \tag{4.20}$$

$$V_{stepn} = V_{step3}\Big|_{A'_1 = \min, A'_2 = \min, A'_3 = \min} \tag{4.21}$$

V_{step4}, V_{step5} … V_{stepn} can be viewed as different cases of V_{step3}. From Fig. 4.39, we can directly get the maximum residue offsets of step4, step5, … ,stepn. So, V_{step3} is the worst case of the proposed method. The maximum residue offset is below

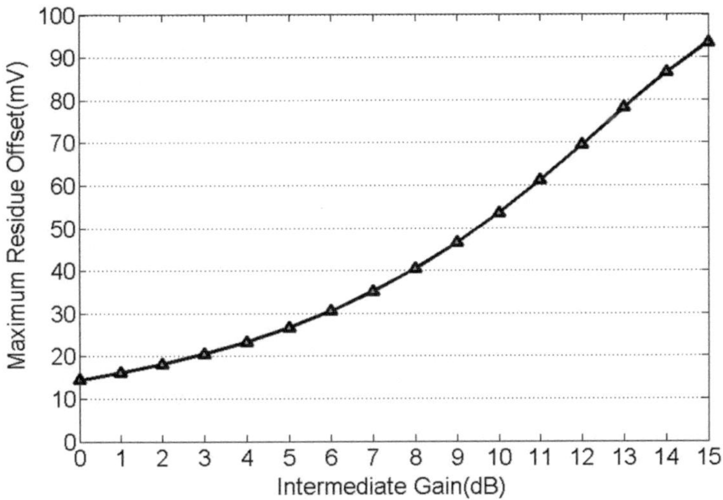

Fig. 4.39 Theoretical maximum residue offsets at different intermediate gains

30 mV when intermediate gain is below 6 dB. Smaller intermediate gain can be used to achieve a smaller residue offset.

To sum up, the presented mixed signal DCOC method is proved to be approximately independent of IF PGA gain. The accuracy of the method mainly rests with the intermediate gain A'_1, A'_2, and A'_3. Figure 4.39 shows the maximum residue output DC offset voltage at different intermediate gains in theory.

4.5.1.3   System Design Considerations

Conventionally, the IF gain of a receiver is arranged for trade-off between the sensitivity and linearity performance of a receiver. In order to get a good sensitivity, the noise figure (NF) should be as low as possible. The noise theory of multistages system shows that a large fore stage gain is good for isolating the poststage noise. As to the receiver chain in Fig. 4.37, the noise of the IF filter is relatively significant. So, the gain of RF part and A_1 are supposed to be enlarged reasonably. For the linearity consideration, large RF gain and A_1 may cause saturation of IF filter when adjacent and alternate channel interference is greater than the desired signal.

With the proposed DCOC method, the arrangement of the IF gain should be optimized for sensitivity, linearity, and the residue DC offset. In part I of the proposed method, A_3 is decreased first, then A_2 is decreased, and A_1 at last. This is good for the NF of the receiver chain but sacrifices the linearity more or less. In part II, A_1, A_2, and A_3 are evenly decreased. This is a commonly used trade-off between noise performance and linearity.

Generally, sensitivity is more significant than linearity for a receiver. The gain arrangement should be optimized for sensitivity on the premise that the linearity requirement is satisfied. The maximum gain of the RF part and PGA1 can be got from the adjacent and alternate channel interference requirements of a specific protocol. The gain of the RF part and PGA1 is supposed to be slightly smaller than its maximum limit and the intermediate gains are suggested to be as small as possible.

4.5.2 DCOC Architecture and Circuit Design

A new DCOC circuit architecture for the zero-IF receiver is presented in this subsection. The architecture adopts the DCOC method introduced in Sect. 4.5.1. The comparator circuit is also given in detail in this part.

4.5.2.1 DCOC Circuit Architecture

A DCOC architecture is shown in Fig. 4.40. Two MUXs and a comparator are used to detect I/Q branch offsets. Six DACs control the offsets of every PGA individually. Memories are adopted to store the calibration results. The calibration process is controlled by digital logic circuits and run only one time when the receiver is just power on.

With the proposed circuit, the calibration process is simplified as shown in Fig. 4.41. As illustrated before, the DCOC method is independent of the IF PGA gain and calibrates at the maximum IF gain. So, the IF gain is set to be maximum while the RF gain is decreased from the maximum to the minimum during the calibration process.

The maximum output offsets of IF PGAs given in Table 4.6 got from Monte Carlo simulation. Maximum output offset of PGA1 consists of PGA1 offset (7 mV) and IF filter offset (5 mV). LSB of DAC is designed to keep the residue offset small and dynamic range of DAC is to overcome the worst case of every PGA.

Offsets produced by self-mixing and leakage of RF circuits are added to the input of PGA1. So, DAC1 calibrates the input of PGA1 to overcome large input offset. DAC2 and DAC3 are designed to confirm the accuracy of calibration.

After the calibration, the control bits of every DAC at different RF gains are stored in the LUT. The calibration results can be directly used when the RF gain changes. So, the setup time of receiver remains small. In this design, the RF gain is in 11 steps from 10 to 40 dB and the IF gain is in 61 steps from 0 to 60 dB.

4.5.2.2 Circuits Design

The comparator circuit is shown in Fig. 4.42. RC filter suppresses the AC signal and high frequency interference. In this design, the minimum IF bandwidth is 500 kHz and the cutoff frequency of RC filter is set to 100 kHz, which cancels the AC signal and consumes small chip area.

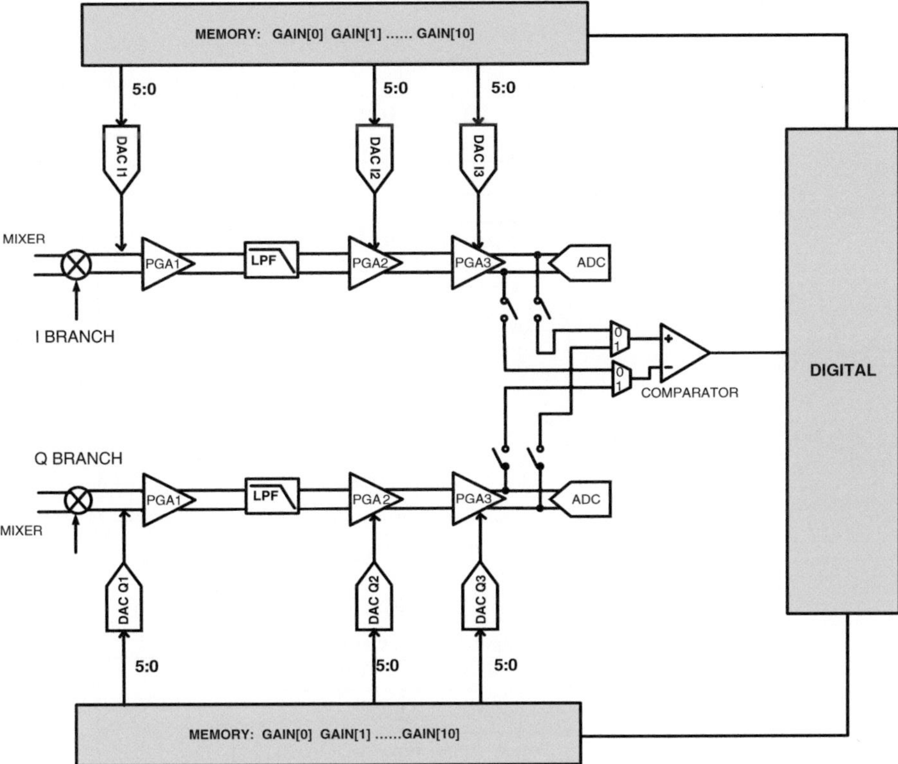

Fig. 4.40 A new DCOC circuit architecture

The comparator adopts a dynamic structure and consumes no DC. The comparison process is controlled by V_{CLK}. When V_{CLK} is low, the comparator is power-off and reset. When V_{CLK} is high, the comparator compares the input voltages. The input referred offset voltage of comparator can affect the precision of the calibration system. It is designed below 0.8 mV.

4.5.3   Measurement Results

The DCOC circuit has been implemented and integrated in the PBS transceiver in the previous section.

Figure 4.43 gives the simulated negative and positive output of I/Q branch PGA3. The waveform of negative and positive output is quite close which means the offset is quite small.

Figure 4.44 gives the measured PGA3 output waveform of one time calibration. The tested waveform matches the simulated waveform well. The DC offset is decreased to be small.

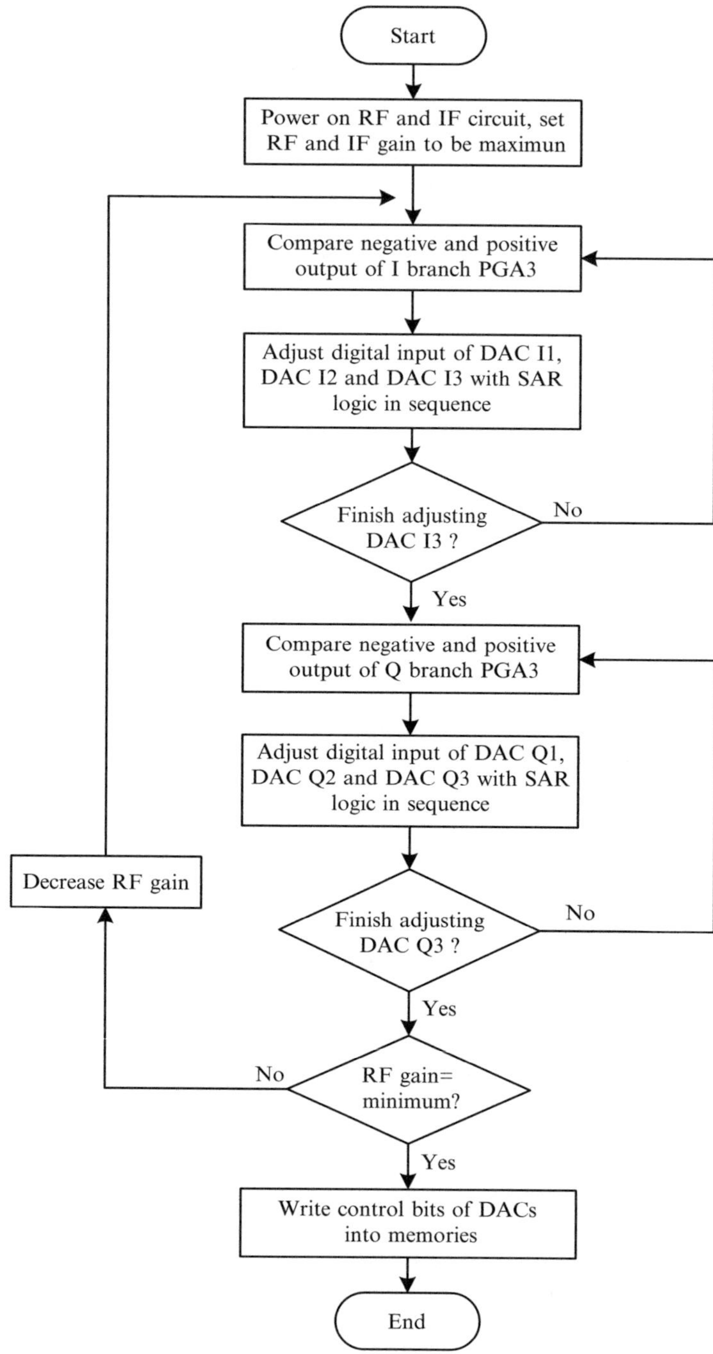

Fig. 4.41 DCOC flowchart

Table 4.6 Offset level and DAC analysis

	PGA1	PGA2	PGA3
Maximum output offset (mV)	12[a]	15	17
Gain (dB)	18	21	21
LSB of correlated DAC (mV)	0.4	2.5	2.5
Dynamic range of correlated DAC (mV)	−12.8–12.4	−80–77.5	−80–77.5
Output offset residue[b] (mV)	3.9	3.3	3.3

[a]Contains the offset of IF filter
[b]With the offset of comparator

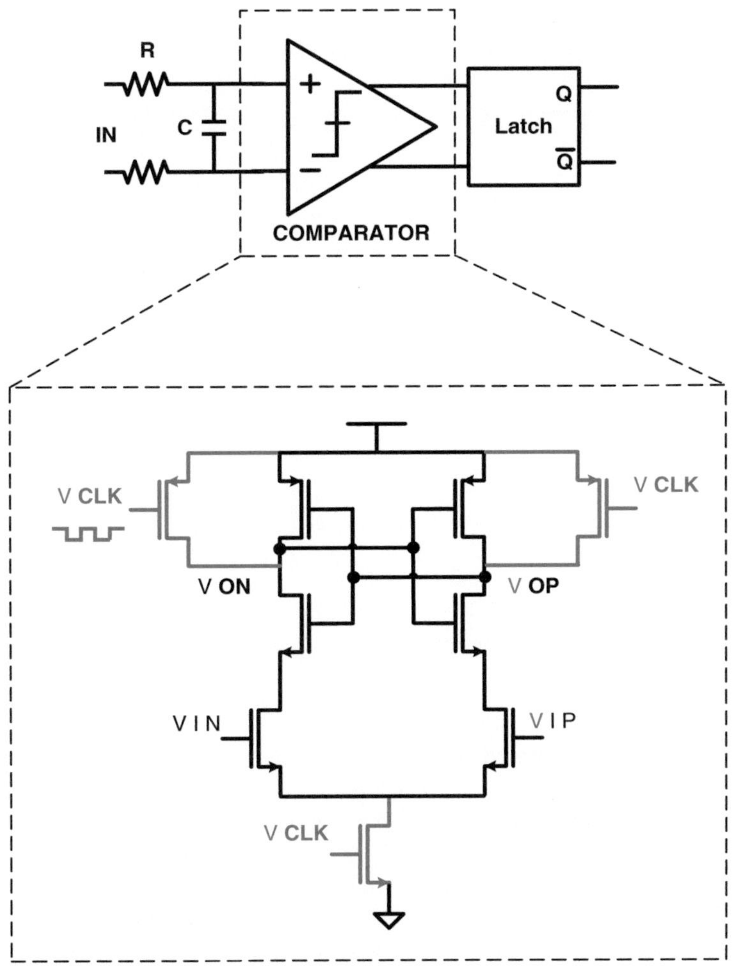

Fig. 4.42 Comparator circuit

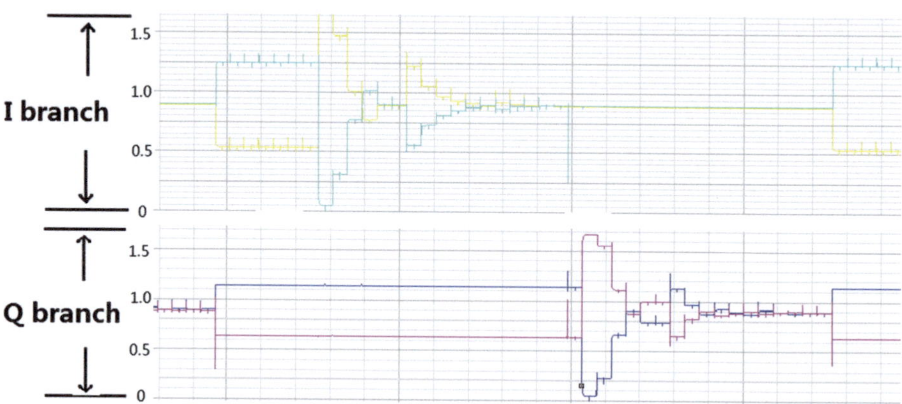

Fig. 4.43 Simulated DC offset voltage during the calibration procedures

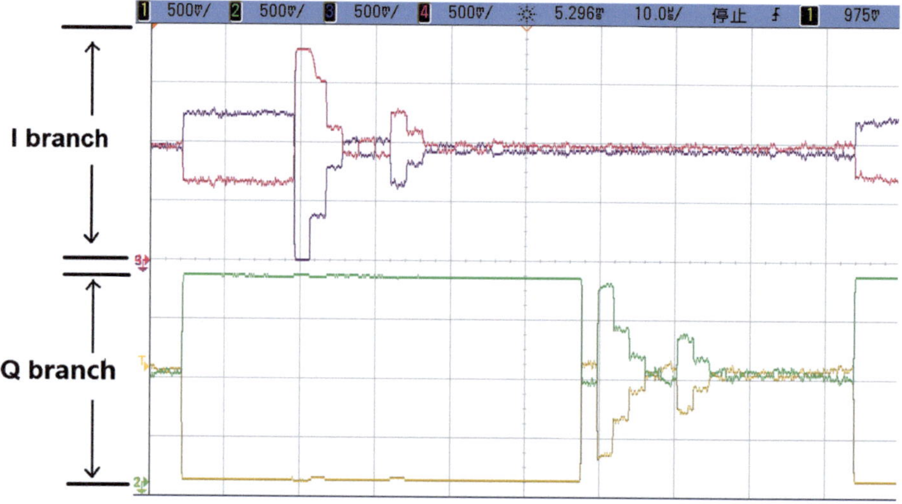

Fig. 4.44 Measured DC offset calibration voltage during the procedures

In this design, the intermediate gains are set to be 14 dB. When the IF gain is changed from 60 to 0 dB, the output residue offset is below 30 mV in most cases. The maximum output residue offset is 63.7 mV and acceptable for the demodulator in the PBS transceiver.

In general, a novel DC offset calibration circuit has been discussed in this section. The DCOC method is designed for the low power zero-IF PBS receiver presented in the previous section. The new DCOC method is independent of the IF gain and requires small die area, which differentiate it from the conventional methods.

References

1. Yoo H-J, Burdett A. ES4: body area network: technology, solutions, and standardization. In: 2011 IEEE international solid-state circuits conference, ISSCC; 2011. p. 531.
2. Wang Z, Jiang H, Xie X, Chen H, Chi B, and Zhang C. Key technologies in the integrated circuit design for the construction of a wireless healthcare system. In: 2011 IEEE international Midwest symposium on circuits and systems, MWSCAS; 2011. p. 1–4.
3. IEEE Computer Society, standard for local and metropolitan area networks—part 15.6: wireless body area networks, IEEE 802 LAN/MAN Standards Committee; 2012. http://www.ieee.org
4. Latré B, Braem B, Moerman I, Blondia C, Demeester P. A survey on wireless body area networks. Wirel Netw. 2010;17:1–18.
5. IEEE Computer Society, standard for information technology—part 15.4: wireless medium access control (MAC) and physical layer (PHY) specifications for low-rate wireless personal area networks (LR-WPANs), IEEE 802 LAN/MAN Standards Committee; 2006. http://www.ieee.org
6. Astrin AW, Bang H. Standardrization for body area networks. IEICE Trans Commun. 2009;92-B:366–72.
7. Bradley PD. Wireless medical implant technology—recent advances and future developments. In: 2011 IEEE European solid-state circuits conference, ESSCIRC; 2011. p. 37–41.
8. Kim S, Lepkowski W, Wilk SJ, Thornton TJ, Bakkaloglu B. A low-power CMOS BFSK transceiver for health monitoring systems. In: 2011 IEEE biomedical circuits and systems conference, BioCAS; 2011. p. 157–60.
9. Wong ACW, Dawkins M, Devita G, Kasparidis N, Katsiamis A, King O, et al. A 1 V 5 mA multimode IEEE 802.15.6/Bluetooth low-energy WBAN transceiver for biotelemetry applications. IEEE J Solid-State Circuits. 2013;48:186–98.
10. Retz G, Shanan H, Mulvaney K, O'Mahony S, Chanca M, Crowley P, et al. A highly integrated low-power 2.4GHz transceiver using a direct-conversion diversity receiver in 0.18um CMOS for IEEE802.15.4 WPAN. In: 2009 IEEE international solid-state circuits conference, ISSCC; 2009. p. 414–5, 415a.
11. Raja MK, Chen X, Lei YD, Zhao B, Yeung BC, Yuan X. A 18 mW Tx, 22 mW Rx transceiver for 2.45 GHz IEEE 802.15.4 WPAN in 0.18-um CMOS. In: 2010 IEEE Asian solid state circuits conference, A-SSCC; 2010. p. 1–4.
12. Kwon Y-I, Park S-G, Park T-J, Cho K-S, Lee H-Y. An ultra low-power CMOS transceiver using various low-power techniques for LR-WPAN applications. IEEE Trans Circuits Syst I Regul Pap. 2012;59:324–36.
13. Borremans J, Mandal G, Giannini V, Debaillie B, Ingels M, Sano T, et al. A 40 nm CMOS 0.4-6 GHz receiver resilient to out-of-band blockers. IEEE J Solid-State Circuits. 2011;46:1659–71.
14. Jiang H, Li F, Chen X, Ning Y, Zhang X, Zhang B, et al. A SoC with 3.9mW 3Mbps UHF transmitter and 240uW MCU for capsule endoscope with bidirectional communication. In: 2010 IEEE Asian solid state circuits conference, A-SSCC; 2010. p. 1–4.
15. Cripps SC. Advanced techniques in RF power amplifier design. London: Artech House; 2002.
16. Kim B, Helman D, Gray PR. A 30-MHz hybrid analog/digital clock recovery circuit in 2-mm CMOS. IEEE J Solid-State Circuits. 1990;25(6):1385–94.
17. Park K, Jeong C, Park J, Lee J, Jo J, Yoo C. Current reusing VCO and divide-by-two frequency divider for quadrature LO generation. IEEE Microw Wirel Compon Lett. 2008;18(6):413–5.
18. Wiser RF, Zargari M, Su DK, Wooley BA. A 5-GHz wireless LAN transmitter with integrated tunable high-Q RF filter. IEEE J Solid-State Circuits. 2009;44:2114–25.
19. Belmas F, Hameau F, Fournier J. A low power inductorless LNA with double Gm enhancement in 130 nm CMOS. IEEE J Solid-State Circuits. 2012;47:1094–103.
20. Tan SC-G, Song F, Zheng R, Cui J, Yao G, Tang L, et al. An ultra-low-cost high-performance Bluetooth SoC in 0.11-um CMOS. IEEE J Solid-State Circuits. 2012;47:2665–77.

21. Kaukovuori J, Stadius K, Ryynanen J, Halonen K. Analysis and design of passive polyphase filters. IEEE Trans Circuits Syst I Regul Pap. 2008;55:3023–37.
22. Zhang L, Jiang H, Li F, Dong J, Cui J, Zhang C, et al. DC offset calibration method for zero-IF receiver removing the PGA-gain-correlated offset residue. AEÜ—Int J Electron Commun. 2013;67:578–84. http://dx.doi.org/10.1016/j.aeue.2012.12.010
23. Gao J, Jiang H, Zhang L, Dong J, and Wang Z. A programmable low-pass filter with adaptive miller compensation for zero-IF transceiver. In: 2012 IEEE international midwest symposium on circuits and systems, MWSCAS; 2012. p. 226–9.
24. Zhang L, Jiang H, Wei J, Dong J, Li W, Gao J, et al. A low-power reconfigurable multi-band sliding-IF transceiver for WBAN hubs in 0.18um CMOS. In: 2010 IEEE Asian solid state circuits conference, A-SSCC; 2012. p. 77–80.
25. Ingels M, Giannini V, Borremans J, Mandal G, Debaillie B, Van Wesemael P, et al. A 5 mm2 40 nm LP CMOS transceiver for a software-defined radio platform. IEEE J Solid-State Circuits. 2010;45:2794–806.
26. Mak P-I, et al. On the design of a programmable-gain amplifier with built-in compact DC-offset cancellers for very low-voltage WLAN systems. IEEE Trans Circuits Syst I Regul Pap. 2008;55(2):496–509.
27. Oh S-M, Park K-S, Yoo H-H, Na Y-S, Kim, T-S. A design of DC offset canceller using parallel compensation. In: IEEE international symposium on circuits and systems, New Orleans; 2007. p. 1685–8.
28. Zheng Y, et al. A CMOS VGA with DC offset cancellation for direct-conversion receivers. IEEE Trans Circuits Syst I Regul Pap. 2008;56(1):103–13.
29. Shih H-Y, et al. A 250 MHz 14 dB-NF 73 dB-gain 82 dB-DR analog baseband chain with digital-assisted DC-offset calibration for ultra-wideband. IEEE J Solid-State Circuits. 2010;45(2):338–50.
30. Lijun Y, et al. A low power mixed signal DC offset calibration circuit for direct conversion receiver applications. J Semiconductors. 2010;32(12):338–50.
31. Razavi B. Design of analog CMOS integrator circuits. New York: McGraw-Hill; 2001.
32. Zhang L, et al. DC offset calibration method for zero-IF receiver removing the PGA-gain-correlated offset residue. AEU—Int J Electron Commun. 2013;67(7):578–84.

Chapter 5
Other Important Circuits

5.1 Power Management

The SID in a wireless medical and health care system is usually powered by miniature coin batteries, the energy and power limit is the most critical constraint in SID design. Thus, the power management system should be carefully designed for the SIDs. Also people are trying to overcome the power constraint by using some other power techniques, such as the wireless energy transfer [1] and energy harvesting techniques. In this chapter, a special energy harvesting technique based on the PZT (piezoelectric ceramic transducer) component will be introduced.

5.1.1 Integrated Power Management Circuit

Battery Life

Before the discussion of the CMOS circuit design techniques, it is quite essential to spend some words on the battery life issue. Actually, the design principle using a miniature coin battery is quite different from other electronic devices powered by batteries with large capacities.

It should be noted that the nominal capacity of a miniature coin battery is usually measured under very small current drain. For instance, the Renata 380 silver-oxide battery manufactured by Renata Batteries has a nominal capacity of 82 mA. This capacity is measured with a 15 kΩ load which means the current drain is only about 100 μA with the 1.55 V nominal voltage [2]. The discharge curve of this battery with a 15 kΩ load is shown in Fig. 5.1.

However, the current consumption of an active SID is usually in the order of milliamperes, and the peak current consumption can reach tens of milliamperes. Both the average current and the peak current are far beyond the nominal discharge current of the coin batteries. With such amount of current drain, the battery capacity will be much less than the nominal values.

Z. Wang et al., *CMOS IC Design for Wireless Medical and Health Care,*
DOI 10.1007/978-1-4614-9503-1_5, © Springer Science+Business Media New York 2014

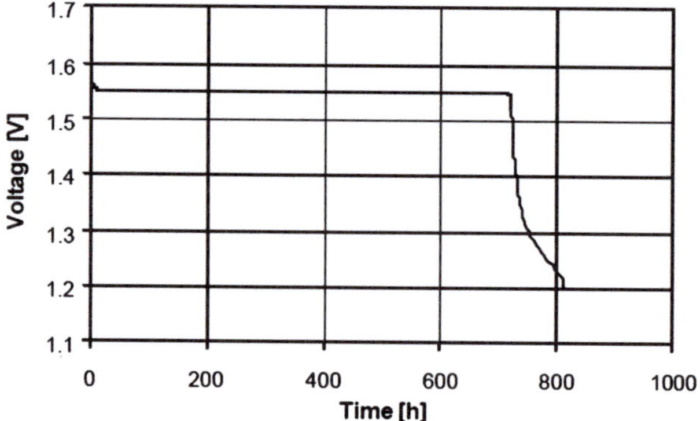

Fig. 5.1 Coin battery nominal discharge curve [2]

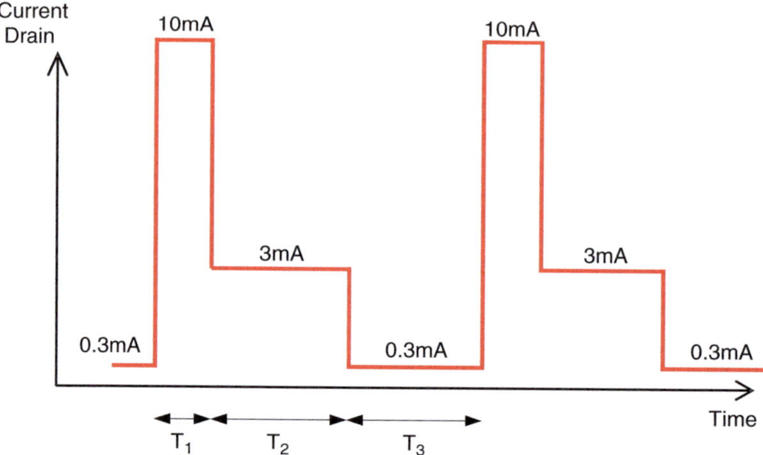

Fig. 5.2 Current curve of a capsule endoscope

To precisely predict the SID battery life, it will be quite critical to measure the real battery life using the actual load current curve. Figure 5.2 shows the current curve of a capsule endoscope. The current curve has a repeat cycle of 0.5 s, and each cycle is divided into three segments, namely T_1, T_2, and T_3, with $T_1=0.06$ s, $T_2=0.23$ s, and $T_3=0.21$ s, respectively. During the experiment, the selected battery (Renata 380) provided power to an emulated load which had the exact current curve as shown in Fig. 5.2. The battery voltage dropped to 1.2 V after 10 h and 37 min. The actual measured capacity is only 28.7 mAh, much less than the nominal value of 82 mAh.

The lesson here is that to precisely predict the battery life for a miniature SID, it will be quite critical to do some experiment on the selected battery using the actual load current curve. The nominal battery life from the datasheet might be misleading due to the difference between the nominal battery current curve and the actual current amplitude.

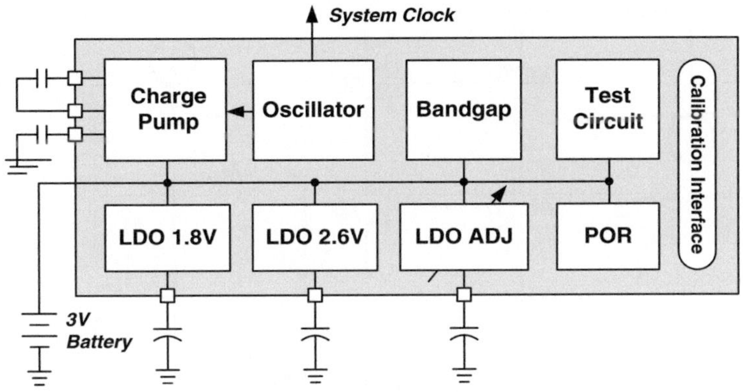

Fig. 5.3 Block diagram of integrated PMU in capsule endoscope chip

Integrated PMU

A wireless medical/health care SID usually is encapsulated in a miniature package, where the PCB area is very limited. That means very few on-board components can be placed. In order to save the PCB area, it is necessary to integrate the power management unit (PMU) with as few on-board components as possible. Moreover, the values of the on-board components such as capacitors should be adequately small to ensure their availability in the micro surface mounted device (SMD) package. Additionally, an effective calibration method should be provided for the PMU as the on-chip resistors and capacitors suffer from the process variation.

The circuit design for an SID integrated PMU will be explained by taking the wireless endoscope capsule as an example, which is powered by two 1.55 V silver-oxide batteries connected in series. The system has several power supply domains including CMOS image sensor analog circuits, RF (Radio Frequency) circuits, digital core, LEDs, and I/O. Conventionally, the supply voltage regulation was realized by a separated PMU chip. However, the miniature requirement of the capsule endoscope raises very stringent demand on the area of PCB board as well as the number of on-board components. The integration of PMU allows one to greatly reduce the on-board components and PCB routing area. Due to the fact that the PMU is integrated, a deep alignment between the performance requirements of the functional blocks and design parameters can be done such as the load capability, voltage tuning, and power supply rejection (PSR). The integration also facilitates the microcontroller to control and calibrate the PMU digitally. The block diagram of the integrated PMU in a capsule endoscope is shown in Fig. 5.3.

The voltage of analog circuit in CMOS image sensor and RF transceiver is supplied by a low-dropout (LDO) regulator with 2.6 V output voltage. Another 1.8 V LDO is used for the digital circuit of image sensor and I/O. The third LDO is an adjustable one, and it supplies the microcontroller with the flexibility of voltage scaling. Though switching DC-DC converter provides higher conversion efficiency

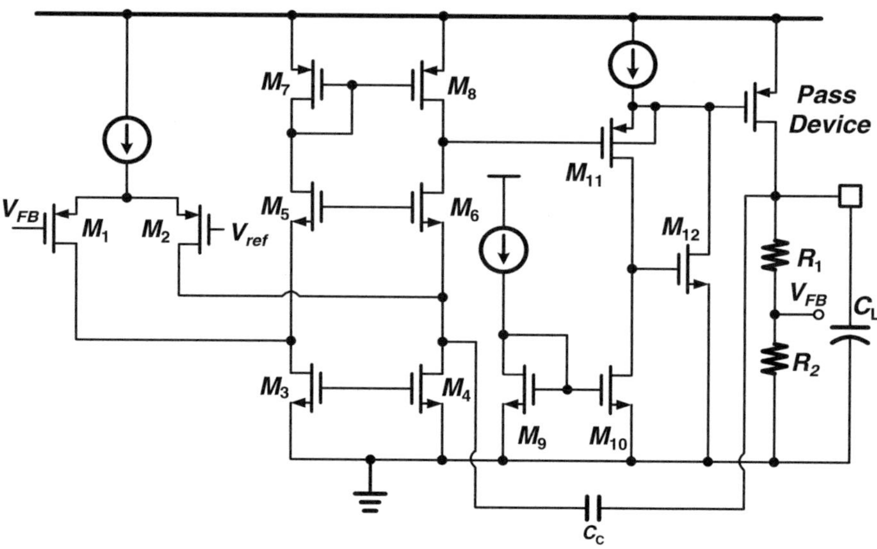

Fig. 5.4 LDO using Ahuja compensation

for low output voltages, several disadvantages have to be considered, such as the large chip area for the complex switching stages, the required off-chip inductor, the large voltage ripple, and the electromagnetic interference (EMI) problem. Moreover, additional noise-reduction filtering has to be utilized to suppress the switching spurious in the receive- and transmit-band for the RF part [3]. Taking these issues into consideration, only linear, LDOs are employed in PMU for voltage regulation.

Low-Dropout Regulator

The LDOs regulate the battery voltage 3 V down to desired output voltages with the trimming capability. Figure 5.4 shows the LDO circuitry design is similar to that in [4]. It is composed of an error amplifier ($M_1 \sim M_8$), a unit-gain buffer ($M_9 \sim M_{12}$) [5], a PMOS pass device, a feedback network (R1, R2), and an off-chip loading capacitance C_L. An Ahuja compensation method [6] is used. The Ahuja compensation exhibits better phase margin across all load levels as well as higher PSR than the classical Miller compensation.

Charge Pump

The capsule endoscope system is equipped with white LEDs as the strobe lights for image capturing. The LEDs need a constant voltage higher than 3 V to provide a constant light density. This is achieved by the integrated charge pump, as shown in Fig. 5.5. The charge pump is actually composed of a voltage doubler and a voltage control feedback loop.

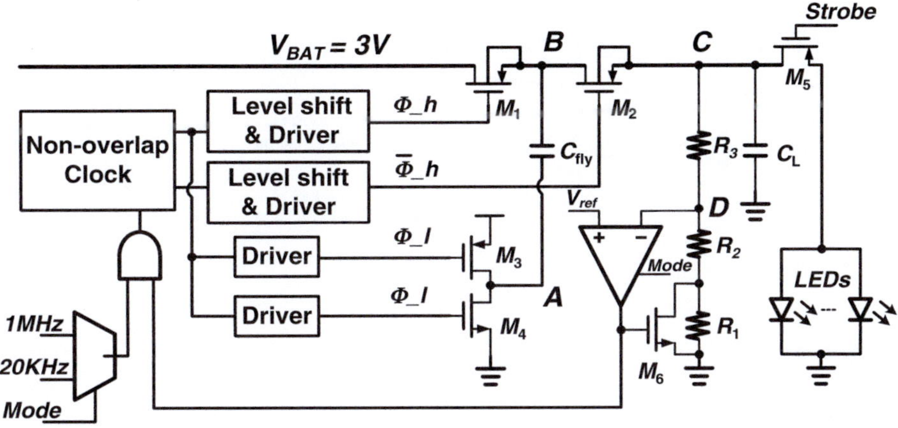

Fig. 5.5 Schematic of charge pump for driving LEDs

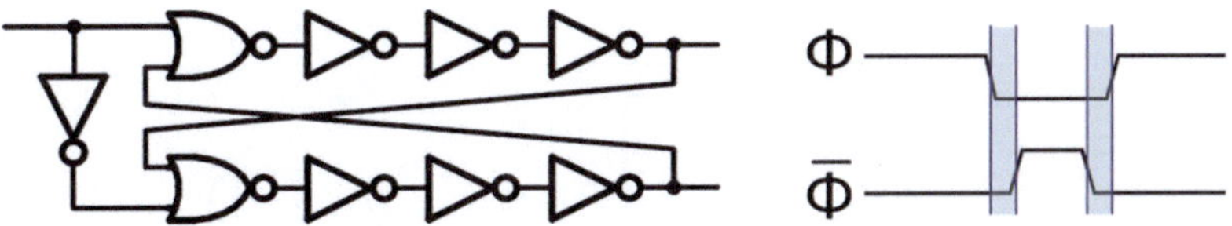

Fig. 5.6 Non-overlapping clock generation circuit

$M_1 \sim M_4$, and the off-chip capacitances C_{fly}, C_L form the voltage doubler. With the non-overlapping clock as shown in Fig. 5.6, the switches $M_1 \sim M_4$ are switched on alternatively such that the two capacitors are charged for voltage doubling. During the clock phase when φ is high, the switches M_1 and M_4 are turned on, the switches M_2 and M_3 are turned off, and the capacitor C_{fly} is charged to V_{BAT}. During the clock phase when $\bar{\varphi}$ is high, the switches M_1 and M_4 are turned off, the switches M_2 and M_3 are turned on, the voltage on node A is charged to V_{BAT}, and the voltage on node B is boosted to about 2 V_{BAT}. The charge on C_{fly} will be moved to C_L until the voltages on these two capacitors are equal. Ideally, the output voltage can be as high as 2 V_{BAT} with this voltage doubler.

It is important to make sure that there is no short current through the switches $M_1 \sim M_4$ during the transitions between the on and off states. The driving circuit for M_3 and M_4 is shown in Fig. 5.7. The input signal to the driving circuit is a single phase clock signal, and the output is a pair of non-overlapping clocks which drive M_3 and M_4, respectively. With the non-overlapping clocks, M_3 and M_4 will never be switched on simultaneously, so that there will be no short current.

The feedback loop in Fig. 5.5 is used to regulate the output voltage to a desired value. To save the energy, two different operating modes are implemented. When the strobe signal is active, the charge pump works in the high speed mode with a high clock frequency together with a large bias current for the feedback loop circuit. In the high speed mode, the charge pump can provide an adequately large current

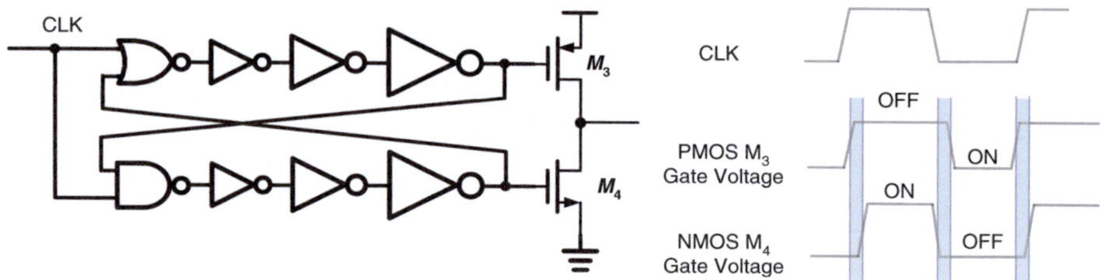

Fig. 5.7 Driving circuit without short current

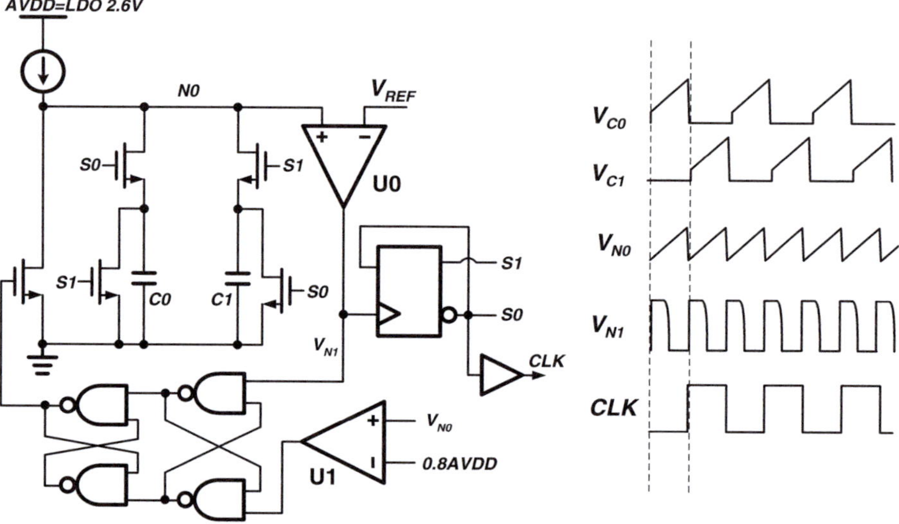

Fig. 5.8 On-chip clock generator and simulated signals

for the strobe LEDs. In the low speed mode without the need of strobe lighting, a
low-frequency clock and a small bias current are sent to the charge pump to maintain the boosted voltage, and the power consumption of the charge pump is notably
lower than that in the high speed mode.

On-Chip Oscillator

An on-chip oscillator is designed to provide clock for the charge pump, the digital
core of the ASIC, and the CMOS image sensor. The oscillator circuit is shown in
Fig. 5.8. Capacitor C0 and C1 are charged and discharged alternatively. By merging
VC0 and VC1, a saw tooth wave is generated at node N0 and then compared to the
reference voltage using a comparator U0 which then outputs a square waveform.
A T flip-flop is driven by the output of U0 to generate a clock signal with 50 %

duty cycle. A second comparator U1 is used to reset the oscillator in case the self-oscillation frequency exceeds the available speed of U0. The oscillator is supplied by an LDO in order to make the frequency independent of the variation of the battery voltage.

5.1.2   Wireless Power Switch

For implantable wireless medical/health care SIDs, such as bladder monitors, pacemakers, and wireless capsule endoscope systems, the implementation of a compact but effective power switch is not trivial. A typical implantable SID is usually sealed in a miniature biocompatible package. For most of today's implantable SIDs, the electrical systems are powered with miniature batteries sealed inside the implantable SIDs, which means the direct power switching is not feasible. An effective wireless power switch is required to shut down the electrical systems before the usage and to power up the electrical systems when the implantable SIDs are prepared for body implantation (swallowing for the case of capsule endoscope systems).

The magnetism stimulated dry reed switch is widely used for implantable SIDs [7, 8]. In such applications, the dry reed switch is sealed inside the implantable SID, and serves as the power switch. However, the dry reed switch-based power switch has many disadvantages. The electromagnet or permanent magnet required to operate the switch adds too much trouble to the production, transportation, and storage. Possible power leakage may shorten the implantable SID product storage time, or even exhaust the batteries before the usage. Furthermore, the dry reed switch cannot be integrated in ICs, and its dimension turns to be one obstacle of the implantable SID size reduction.

In this subsection, an IC-based wireless power switch will be presented which can be used to replace the dry reed switches in implantable SIDs. The major function of this switch IC is to receive RF signals which contain switch operation commands, and then to control the power of the entire implantable SID accordingly. Since this IC is based on the wireless energy recovery, it consumes zero standby current when serving as the power switch. Wireless identification is also adopted to make this switch immunized from space noises and disturbances. The presented IC-based power switch can eliminate the troubles associated with the magnetism required to operate the dry reed switch. And it also features the excellent compatibility with implantable SID main ICs.

Wireless Power Switch Architecture

The dry reed switch-based power switching for implantable SIDs will be briefly reviewed. And then the proposed power switch and the switch IC architecture will be introduced.

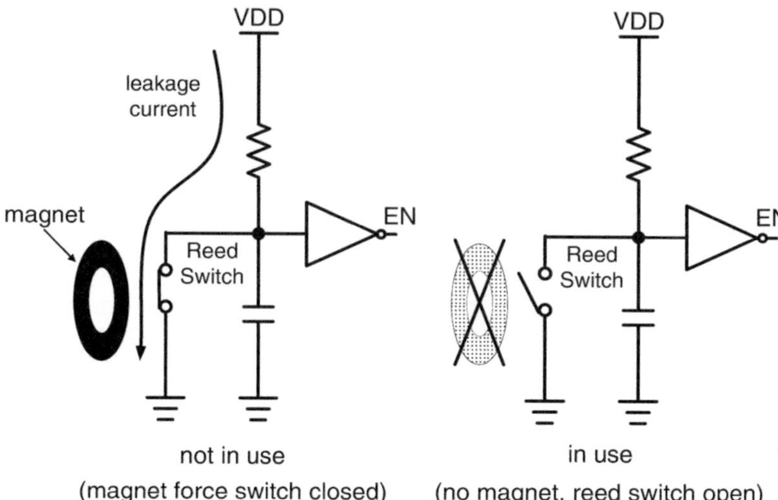

Fig. 5.9 Power switching using a dry reed switch

For a typical implantable SID such as the capsule endoscope system which uses a dry reed switch, a permanent magnet or an electromagnet has to be used to differentiate the implantable SID power on/off states. More specifically, the implantable SID is powered off if the magnet is put close enough, and it is powered on when the magnet is removed. However, the available ultra-miniature dry reed switches usually have normally open contacts, such as the RI-80 series dry reed switch provided by Coto Technology. In other words, when the implantable SID is not in usage, the magnet is put close to it, and the dry reed switch is actually closed. This means the dry reed switch cannot be directly used as the power switch. Instead, it is used to generate a system enable signal. Figure 5.9 shows how the system enable signal is generated with the aid of a pull-up resistor and an inverter. It is clear that when implantable SID is not in use, there is a current leakage path through the pull-up resistor and the dry reed switch. For an implantable SID powered by miniature batteries, such kind of leakage current is the major limit factor of the product storage time. This is one major disadvantages of the dry reed switch-based power switching, in addition to the added complexity and the increased product size.

To overcome the disadvantages associated with the dry reed switch-based power switching, an IC-based wireless power switch is proposed. Figure 5.10 shows a block diagram of the power switch for a wireless capsule endoscope system. In this power switch, a dedicated switch IC, the most import part of this work, receives 915 MHz RF signals containing an identification code and the switching command. The switch IC recovers energy from the received RF signals, and supplies most of the internal blocks inside this IC. This switch IC then generates an enable/disable signal as requested by the switching command, and this enable/disable signal is

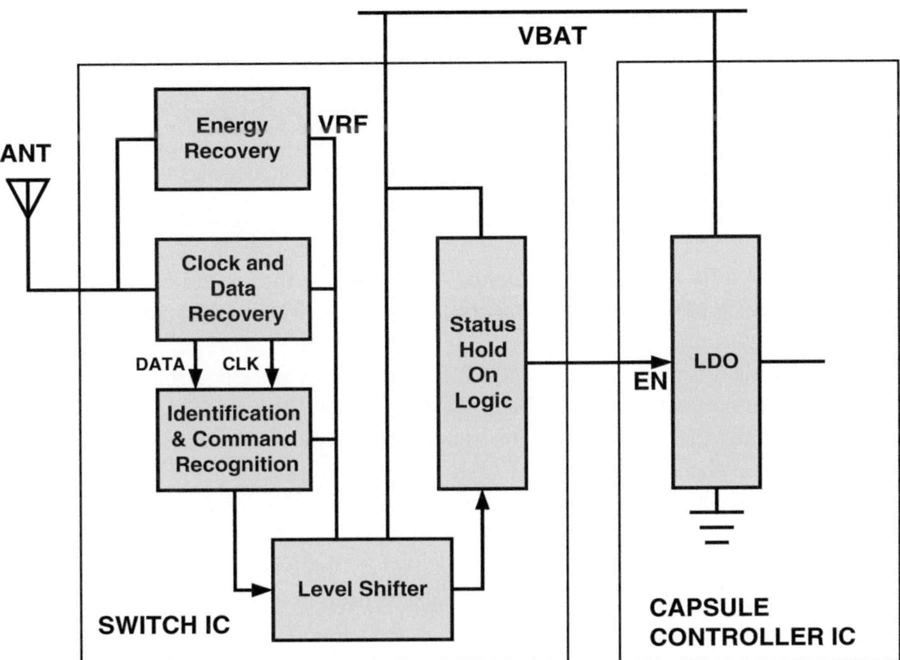

Fig. 5.10 Wireless power switch architecture

used to control an LDO linear regulator inside the capsule controller IC. In this sense, the LDO serves as the switch device of the whole switch system, while the wireless switch IC can be viewed as the control part of this switch system. A receiving antenna is required for the system to work.

The function blocks in the switch IC are described as follows. The energy recovery block converts part of the incoming RF signal power to a dc voltage (VRF), and stores it on an on-chip capacitor. This dc voltage supplies all active circuits in this IC except the status-hold-on-logic block and the level shifter. The clock and data recovery (CDR) block recovers a digital signal from the received RF signal with amplitude shift keying (ASK) modulation, and it also generates a synchronous clock simultaneously for the next block. The identification and command recognition (ICR) block is an all digital block. This block handles the output from the CDR block, such as cyclic redundancy checks (CRC), according to the communication protocol. This block compares the received device identification code to the identification code stored locally to check if a valid device ID has been received. It also recognizes valid switching command. When a valid command with a right ID is received, the ICR block outputs a pulse. The level shifter that follows the ICR block converts the pulse voltage level from VRF to the battery level V_{BAT} for further interfacing with the LDO supplied by implantable SID batteries. The rising edge of the pulse will toggle the enable/disable signal, and hence the implantable SID electrical

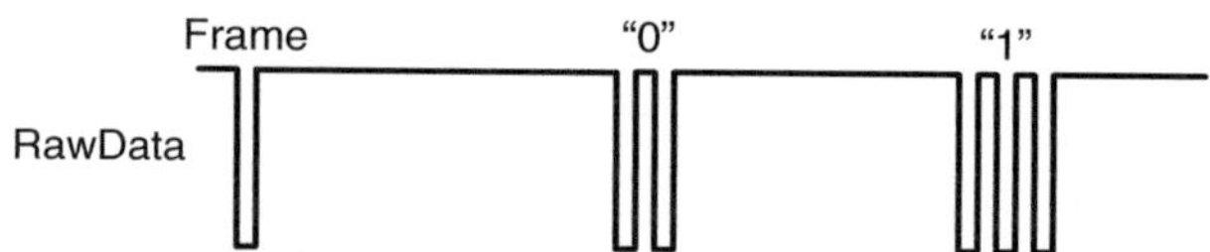

Fig. 5.11 Communication coding scheme for wireless switch

system powered by the LDO is switched on/off. Inside the switch IC, those circuit blocks connected to the batteries only contain a few logic gates and consume almost zero standby current.

Since the data transmission needed for switching operation is not very complicated, the communication protocol can also be simple. The carrier is set to 915 MHz which falls into the ISM band. The modulation type chosen is On-Off Keying (OOK) which is the simplest kind of ASK. The bit rate is set to 25 kbps. The system is designed to tolerate a certain variation in the carrier frequency and the data rate. Figure 5.11 shows the data coding scheme. Bit "0" is represented by two consecutive negative pulses, while bit "1" is represented by three pulses. The pulse width is 1 μs nominally. In addition, one negative pulse is used to define the start and the end of a data frame.

A valid data frame is composed of a 7-bit command section and a 16-bit ID section. Each section is followed by a 6-bit CRC code. For the time being, only one command (on/off toggling) is implemented in the switch IC to control the LDO in the controller IC. The command sets can be expanded if needed in the future. Note that a 16-bit ID is used for this switch system, and this long ID will greatly lower the risk that the switch is turned on/off by some disturbance signal in the 915 MHz ISM band.

Circuits Design

The design details of the major function blocks in the switch IC will be presented.

Energy Recovery

A multistage rectifier is used to convert the received 915 MHz RF power into a dc power supply stored on a 300 pF on-chip capacitor. The rectifier has a structure of Dickson voltage multiplier [9]. This kind of circuit needs low threshold diodes or MOSFETs. The Schottky barrier diode has been often used due to its low threshold voltage and good high-frequency response [10].

Figure 5.12 is the schematic of the rectifier using Schottky diode in the switch IC. D1–D8 are Schottky junctions, and D9–D11 are normal PN junctions. The Schottky diodes and capacitors form a rectifier which converts RF power to dc supply, while

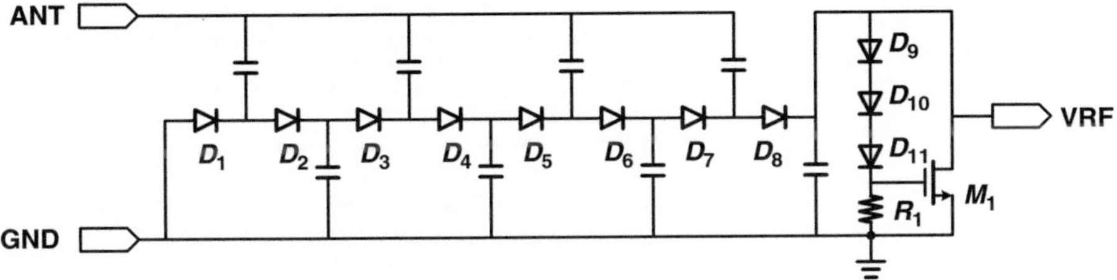

Fig. 5.12   Schematic of the energy recovery block for dc supply

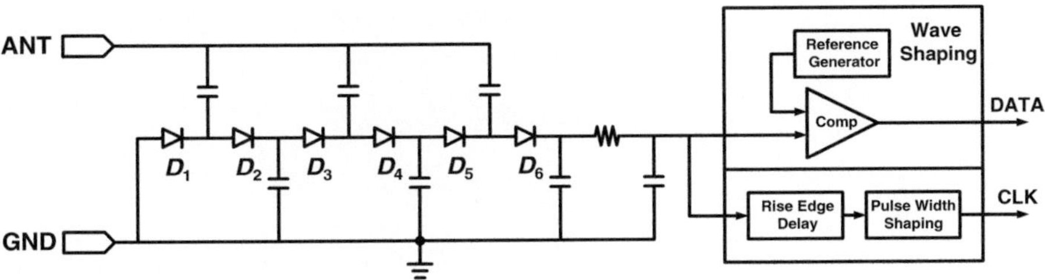

Fig. 5.13   Schematic of clock and data recovery block

the normal diodes, the resistor, and the MOSFET form a voltage regulator which limits the highest level of dc supply.

As Schottky diode is not available in most commercial standard CMOS process, which is also the same for this case, the Schottky diode has been implemented with some special layout design [11]. For this customized Schottky diode, the interface between the metal and the low-doped n-well forms a Schottky junction. The metal is the anode of the diode, while the n-well is the cathode. The saturation current is determined by the size of the contact, which is 5 μm by 5 μm.

Clock and Data Recovery Block

The CDR block demodulates the baseband digital signal from the RF carrier. It is combined by envelop detection circuit, wave-shaping circuit, and clock regeneration circuit, as shown in Fig. 5.13. The envelope detection circuit filters the RF carrier and restores the signal envelope. It also uses the Dickson voltage multiplier structure as shown in Fig. 5.12, though the stage number is reduced to 3. The wave-shaping circuit is basically a comparator which reshapes the RF envelope to a standard logic signal. The logic signal is then buffered and input to the digital block. The clock signal is regenerated also from the RF envelope signal with the aid of a rising edge delay cell and a pulse width shaping circuit.

Fig. 5.14 Micrograph of the
wireless switch IC

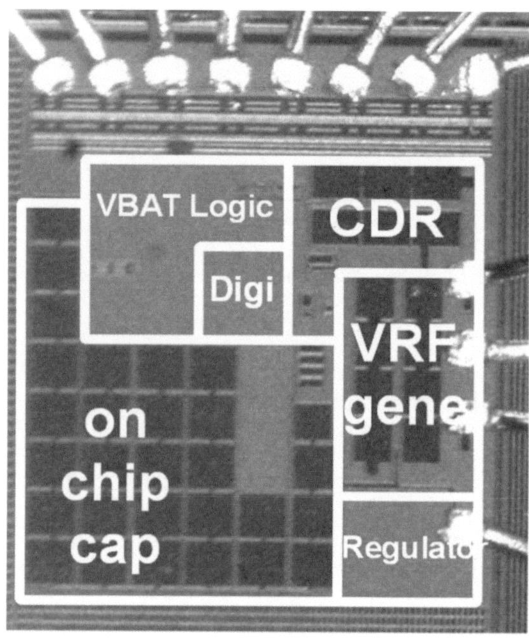

Identification and Command Recognition

This digital block is used to check the received ID code and recognize the command
code. In order to distinguish command source, the switch system has a 16-bit ID.
A certain switch can only be operated by an RF signal with a matching ID code.
In the work flow, the digital block does not respond until it receives a valid command followed by a matching ID. The technology used for this IC does not support
EEPROM, and as a substitute, the ID of each switch is determined by ID pins connected to high or low externally. Though the switch system supports 16-bit ID code,
only four ID pins are used in this implementation due to die area limitation. These
four ID pins corresponds to 16 different IDs. Sixteen 16-bit pseudo random codes
are chosen to represent these 16 IDs. It is anticipated that the switch system can
have adequate disturbance immunity with 16-bit ID codes.

Measurement Results

The switch circuit was implemented in 0.18 μm Mixed-Mode CMOS technology.
Figure 5.14 is the micrograph of the die. The die area is 0.94 mm by 0.95 mm.

Direct measurements have been carried out on this IC using the chip-on-board
assembly. These measurements check how the energy recovery circuit works.
Different input RF power levels from a network analyzer have been injected into
the ANT pin of the switch IC. The injected RF power level generates at least
1 V at VRF node which is the minimum limit for the other circuit block to work.

Table 5.1 Switch IC input port measurement results using network analyzer

Network analyzer output power (dBm)	SWR	Actual received signal power (μW)	VRF (V)
−4.5	15.0	41.7	1.0
−3.3	11.6	63.9	1.2
−1.9	5.9	116.2	1.4
−0.2	5.7	237.6	1.6
1.5	4.1	436.2	1.8

Table 5.2 Wireless switch IC performance summary

Technology	0.18 μm Standard CMOS
Die area	0.94 × 0.95 mm
RF frequency	915 MHz ± 10 MHz
Minimum RF input power	40 μW
Energy recovery load capability	2.7 μA @ 60 μW input
Modulation	OOK
Data rate	25 kbps
Standby current	<10 nA

The actual RF power received at the ANT pin is much less than the output of the analyzer due to port impedance mismatch. However, the actual received power can be calculated using (5.1). In this equation, PIN is the output power of the analyzer, while PR is the actual received RF power at the ANT pin. SWR stands for the standing wave ratio which can be read from the analyzer.

$$P_R = P_{IN}\left[1 - \left(\frac{SWR-1}{SWR+1}\right)^2\right] \tag{5.1}$$

Table 5.1 shows how the recovered DC supply voltage VRF changes with different input RF signal levels. It can be found that switch IC can work with an RF input power of ~40 μW minimally. The driving capability of the energy recovery circuit has been measured by applying an external to VRF node. The measurement shows that energy recovery can supply at least 2.7 μA current to an external load when the ANT port received an RF power of ~60 μW. However, the variation in SWR indicates that the impedance of the ANT port varies with input RF signal power. This might bring difficulty to design the receiving antenna for the switch IC.

The standby current consumption from the batteries has been directly measured. This standby current is always below 10 nA and can almost be neglected compared to the several μA standby current consumed by the dry reed switch case.

Table 5.2 summaries the wireless power switch IC.

Function Verification

The wireless power switch IC has been packed into a real wireless endoscope capsule for verification. The switch IC uses a spiral metal line (3 cm long when straightened)

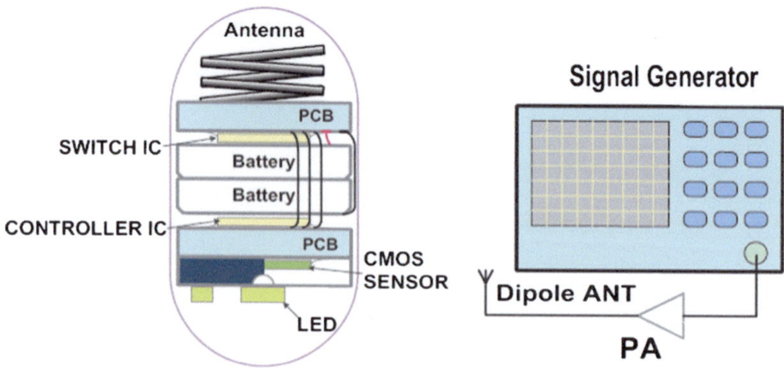

Fig. 5.15 A wireless endoscope capsule with the power switch IC

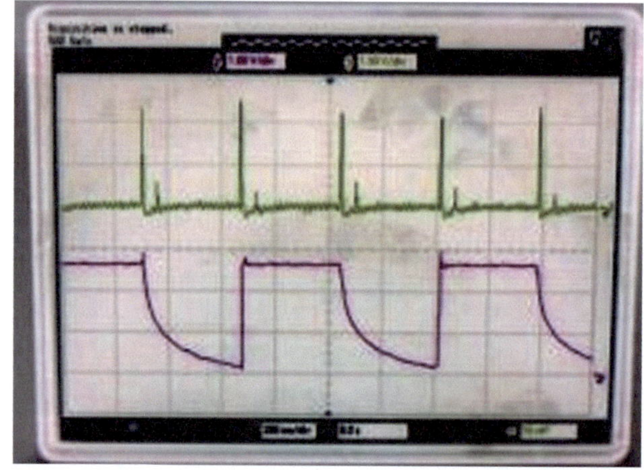

Fig. 5.16 Oscilloscope waveforms for endoscope system verification using the wireless power switch IC (*upper*: envelope of 915 MHz switching command; *lower*: endoscope LDO output)

as its antenna. Figure 5.15 shows the capsule verified. A signal generator feeds 915 MHz RF signal with switching commands to a dipole antenna.

During verification, the signal generator sends out a periodical switching command modulated on 915 MHz. The oscillator waveforms are shown in Fig. 5.16. It can be seen clearly that the LDO in the capsule controller IC toggles with the received RF signal containing the switching command.

Figure 5.17 shows the endoscope capsule in whole. In this figure, the LDO in the capsule has been turned on wirelessly through the power switch IC, and the white LEDs inside the capsule have already been ignited.

In summary, the wireless power switch IC is designed for the implantable SIDs. This power switch IC is proposed to substitute the dry reed switch-based power switching used widely in today's implantable SIDs. Compared to the dry reed

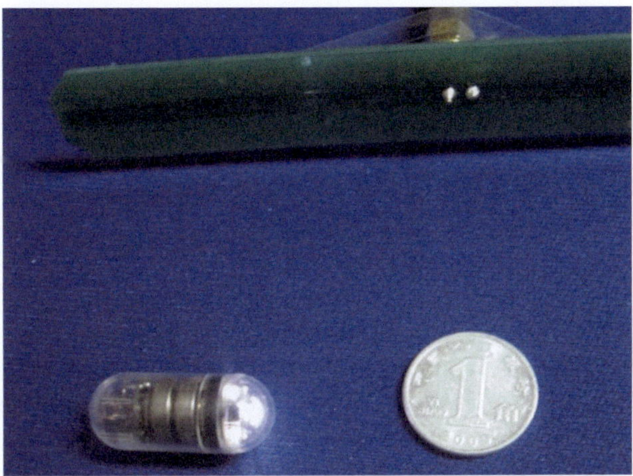

Fig. 5.17 Wireless endoscope capsule switched on wirelessly (*upper*: dipole antenna sending switching commands)

switch, this new power switch can be easily integrated with other ICs inside the implantable SIDs. It can help to reduce implantable SID production and usage complexity, alleviate the power leakage, and reduce the size of implantable SIDs. The wireless identification technology adopted in this power switch IC can help to reduce implantable SID switch malfunction due to electromagnetic disturbance.

5.1.3   Power Harvesting from PZTs

The limited lifetime and the physical dimensions of miniature wireless medical/ health SIDs result in the demand of new power source other than the traditional batteries, especially for some power-critical or maintenance-free real-time implantable SIDs, such as the implantable wireless sensors and orthopedic implants etc. Since the electrical energy can be converted from ambient energy (e.g., thermal energy, mechanical energy), the power generation from ambient energy has received considerable attention. In the field of mechanical energy transformation, piezoelectric materials have been of great interest. Various analysis and approaches of energy harvesting using piezoelectric materials have been reported [12–20]. Some researcher have been focusing on the characteristic of power generation of piezoelectric material [12–14] while some others are investigating power optimization and the electrical interface circuit of power generation [15, 16].

In [14], PZT wafers and flexible, multilayer polyvinylidene fluoride (PVDF) films are used inside shoes to convert mechanical walking energy into usable electrical energy. This system is ultimately able to provide continuously 1.3 mW at 3 V when walking at a pace rate of 0.8 pace/s. The desirable characteristics of piezoelectric

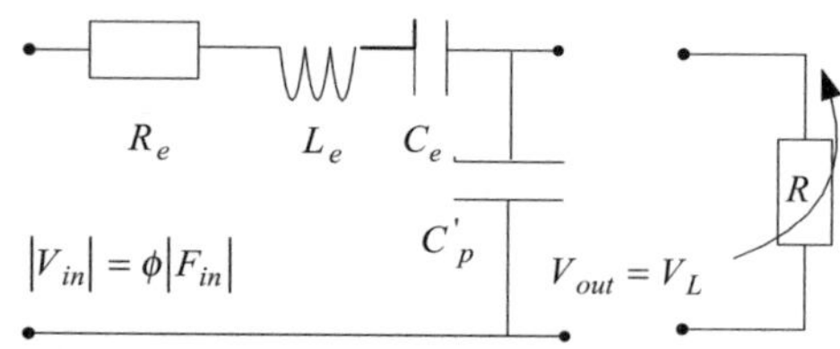

Fig. 5.18 Equivalent circuit of a PZT element

materials for wearable e-textiles are described in [15]. In [16], piezoelectric films are used to extract electrical energy from mechanical vibration in machines to drive MEMS devices. Similarly, more energy (approximately 70 μW) is obtained from machine and building vibrations in [17]. In [18], electricity generation from pressure variations in microhydraulic systems by using piezoelectric materials is studied, yet this work is still on the conceptual level. Flexible piezoelectric polymers could also be used to convert oceanic flow into electric power [19]. Unregulated energy is used in [20], where a theoretical analysis of power generation using PZT is presented. Several important considerations in designing such generators are explored. Finally, an application is presented where electrical energy is generated inside a prototype Total Knee Replacement (TKR) implant.

In contrast to [20], the technique discussed in this section aims to use self-powered sensors in real-world clinical implants. Compared to [20], smaller PZT elements can be used with the presented technique, which specifically addresses the problem of limited space available inside an implant. Hence a more practical application scenario is presented. The main contributions of the presented work are as follows:

1. Smaller PZT elements are used with a volume of only $0.5 \times 0.5 \times 1.8$ cm^3 (compared to $1 \times 1 \times 1.8$ cm^3 in [20]).
2. A comprehensive experimental framework for PZT elements has been established. Designers could use this framework to evaluate major design tradeoffs in PZT-based system design.
3. The PZT elements designed in this work has been deployed in an embedded monitoring system, which has been implemented with a commercial EDA toolkit. Some modules including the power circuit, RF (Radio Frequency) circuit were already taped out in 0.18-μm CMOS process.

PZT Modeling

To design an energy harvesting circuit, the PZT component modeling should be carried out first. The relationships between mechanical stress and strain and electric field and electrical displacement (charge per unit area) and the techniques used to measure piezoelectric material properties were standardized in the IEEE Standard on piezoelectricity [21]. The equivalent electronic circuit of a PZT element is shown in Fig. 5.18 and an analysis can be found in [20].

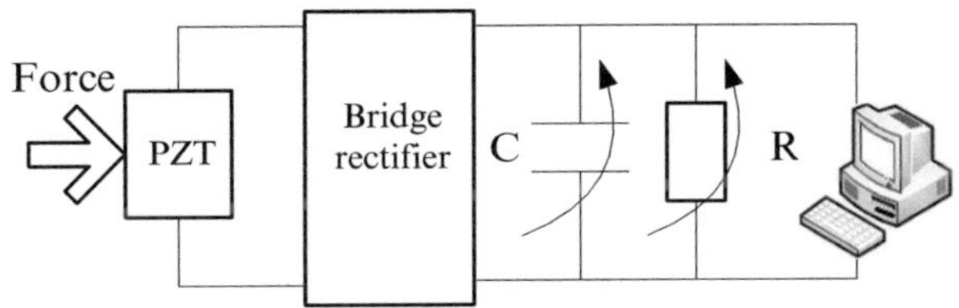

Fig. 5.19 PZT energy harvesting experiment with one PZT

Experimental System

In the application of TKR for which the PZT energy harvesting will be used, the implant kinematics require the deflection of the bearing surfaces to be small (<10 μm), besides, the usable space inside implants is also extremely limited. Therefore, stiff PZT elements ("TS18-H5-104" from Piezo Systems [20, 22]) are used in this work.

First of all, the amount of power that can be generated by a single PZT needs to be determined. Besides, as the integrated circuit will be the load of PZT element, the relationship between the load of the PZT element and the power also needs to be established. According to [20], piezoelectric materials at low frequencies are essentially purely capacitive devices. One method to store energy is to include a rectifier to convert the bipolar piezoelectric output into a unipolar signal, and a capacitor in parallel with the resistive load. When the storage capacitance is equivalent to the equivalent capacitance of the PZT element, the maximum power can be obtained [20].

The experimental circuit shown in Fig. 5.19 includes five components, namely a PZT element, a bridge rectifier, an adjustable load resistor (R), and a adjustable storage capacitor (C), and a computer to generate specific force waveforms which are applied on the PZT. Force magnitude, PZT displacement, and voltage measurements through a 12-bit data acquisition card (National Instruments 6025E [20]) are recorded using *LabView* as the user interface. The force on PZT is applied directly using a single-axis *Mini-Bionix MTS (858)* machine. The International Standards Organization (ISO) force waveform (ISO 14243-1, 2002) is used to simulate the typical axial forces on TKR implants [13]. In this work, the 31 mode of operation is used [20].

The experimental results are obtained by subjecting piezoelectric elements to various cyclic mechanical loads using a single-axis *Mini-Bionix* test machine. This machine is equipped with a PID (Proportional-Integral-Derivative) controller and is capable of applying arbitrary force or displacement waveforms to the PZT elements. In the experiments, the values of the capacitance and of the resistance are adjusted within the range of 0.1 pF~100 μF and 100 Ω~1 MΩ, respectively. The experimental result of the average power output values of the resistor R and capacitor C over a series of repeated loading cycles is shown in Fig. 5.20.

In Fig. 5.20, two peak power values can be identified. The first peak appears when the resistance R is within the range of 10~20 kΩ and when the capacitance C is within the range of 0.2~100 nF. The second peak appears with R and C within the

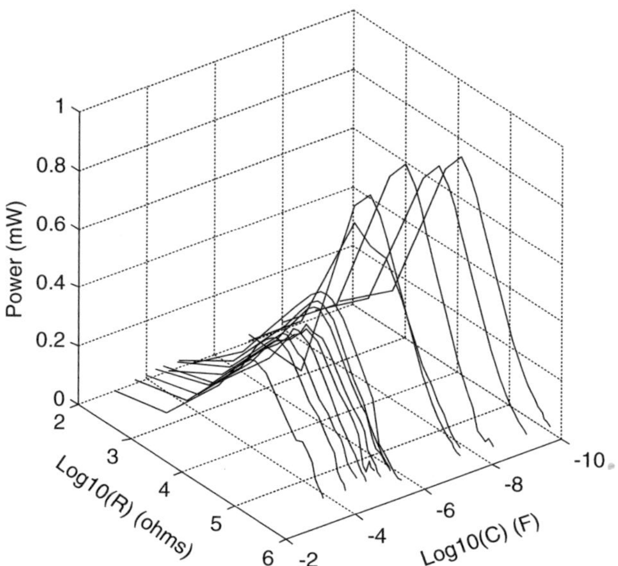

Fig. 5.20 Relationship between power, resistance R, and capacitance C

ranges of 20~50 kΩ and >10 μF, respectively. The values of the two peaks are approximately 800 and 460 μW, respectively. At the first peak, C is very small. As a result, the output ripple in the time domain is much bigger than that of the second peak point. Considering the power circuit design, a smaller ripple is desired.

PZT Model Parameters Fitting

In order to determine the parameters in the equivalent electronic circuit (Fig. 5.18), the second set of experiments is conducted using low-frequency (1 Hz) sinusoidal input force waveforms with amplitudes of 900 N. The experimental circuit is similar with what is shown in the Fig. 5.19 except that the load of the PZT element is only an adjustable resistor in parallel. A nonlinear least square fitting was performed. The fitting results are as follows: $\phi = 0.03$, $L_e = 6 \times 10^{-6} H$, $R_e = 0.4\Omega$, $C_e = 0.77 \times 10^{-6} F$, and $C_p = 01.491 \times 10^{-6} F$. HSPICE is used to simulate the circuit shown in Fig. 5.18, using the fitted parameters. Figure 5.21 shows the average power generated by a single PZT with load R (the circles represent the experimental data and the solid lines represent the simulation results). It can be seen that the accordance of data is very good.

The simulation result shows that much more power that can be transferred to load R when the capacitance is very small and when the load resistance matches the impendence of the power source. This result agrees with the experimental results of the second peak point shown in Fig. 5.20. To minimize output ripple, a larger capacitance (about 10 μF) will be used in the future work.

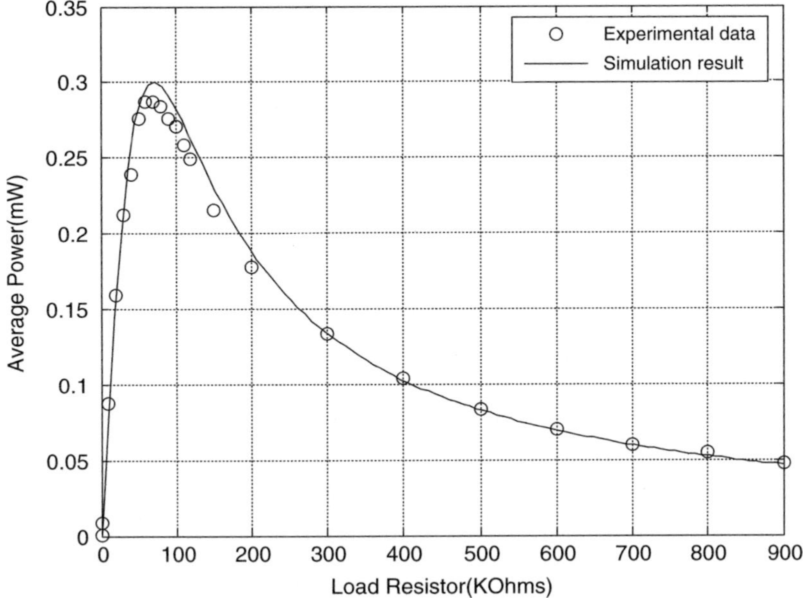

Fig. 5.21 The average power transferred to load R by one PZT

From these results, it can be seen that the simulation data agrees very well with the experimental data, which confirms the fitting parameters. However, the output power generated by a single PZT is rather weak (about 0.3 mW). In order to increase the power output, a third set of experiments is performed with four identical PZT elements connected in parallel. Figure 5.22 shows the average power generated by the four PZTs with load R. Again, the circles represent experimental data, and the solid lines represent the simulation results of the equivalent circuit. The two sets of data match well except for the peak power. The experimental peak power is not four times as much as the peak power generated by a single PZT element. This discrepancy can be explained by the fact that the four PZTs receive different amount of force in the experiments, therefore not every PZT can generate the maximum power (about 0.3 mW), as a result, the power generated by the four PZTs is less than 1.2 mW.

Power Conversion Efficiency

Using the fitting result presented above, the relationship between the efficiency and the frequency and the load R can be calculated. The surface of Fig. 5.23 represents the result for the overall electromechanical efficiency for the raw power produced by the piezoelectric element. The input force profile was sinusoidal with a 900 N amplitude, and the efficiency was calculated for a range of frequencies and load resistors. The results indicate that the best efficiencies are obtained when the frequency is about 79 kHz and when the load is about 89 kΩ. The efficiency peaks as

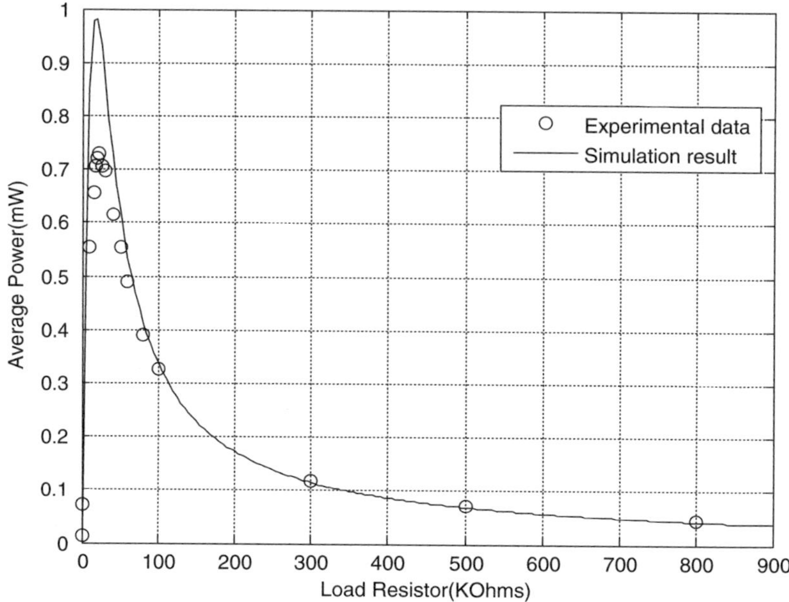

Fig. 5.22 Average power of load R with four PZTs

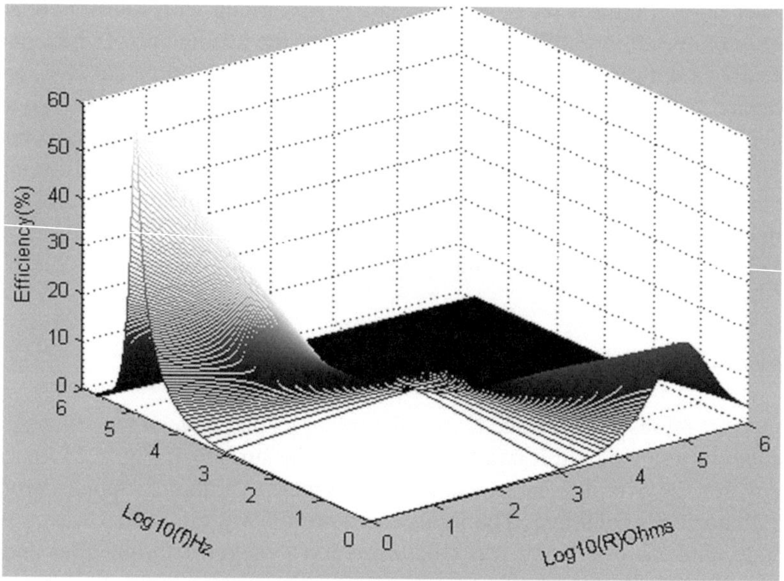

Fig. 5.23 PZT conversion efficiency vs. frequency and resistive load

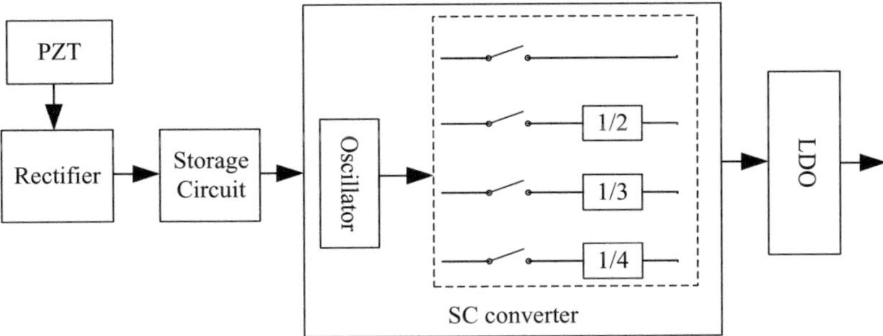

Fig. 5.24 PZT energy harvesting structure

would be expected at the resonant frequency of about 79 kHz in this case. As the input frequency increases, the maximum efficiency occurs at smaller load resistance. That's because as the frequency increases the impedance will decrease. The results are similar to that in [13].

Although motion frequency of patients will be far less 79 kHz when the PZT elements are embedded into orthopedic implants, in other words, we will have to make the PZT elements work at a frequency with lower power conversion efficiency. Nonetheless, we still could maintain a reasonable level of power supply by properly choosing load capacitance and resistance values (R and C within the ranges of 20~50 KΩ and >10 µF respectively).

Energy Harvesting Circuit Design

The proposed PZT energy harvesting structure is shown in Fig. 5.24. In Fig. 5.24, the power generated by PZT is first rectified by a full-wave bridge rectifier to convert the bipolar piezoelectric output to a unipolar output. Then, a capacitor is used as storage element in parallel with the load circuit. An oscillation circuit is embedded to generate clock signals for an "SC converter" (Switching Capacitor based on DC-DC Converter), which will lower the input voltage from approximately 10 to 2 V. The input voltage is controlled by four programmable switches, as shown in the dashed block in Fig. 5.24. Therefore, the power circuit can provide four different voltages to other circuits. Finally, an LDO voltage regulator reduces the voltage further to a steady value around 1.5 V.

The power harvesting circuit is shown in Fig. 5.25. The switched capacitor (SC) converter is used to regulate the charged capacitor supply from 1.8 to 0.8 V, and the LDO is used to regulate the 0.8 V output voltage to 0.3~0.6 V. The SC converter can perform several ratios of step-down functions, such as 1, 2/3, 1/2, and 1/3. All of these different functions use a same capacitors' topology, which will be set to different topologies according to different step-down voltage ratios, as shown in Fig. 5.26. The "Variable step-down ratio switched capacitor converter [21]" provides the scaling voltages according to the control signals generated by the "Step-down

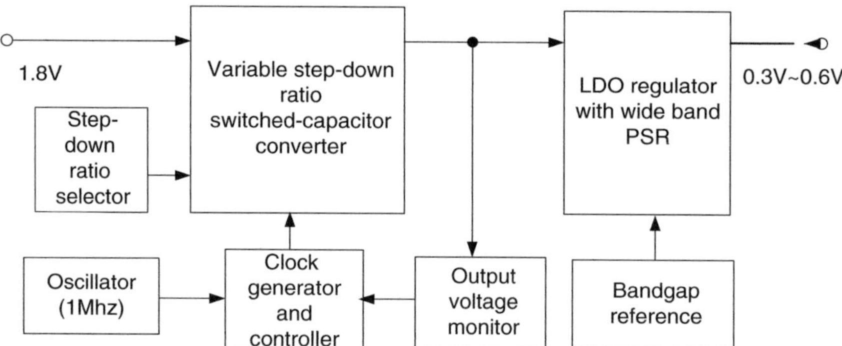

Fig. 5.25 Power harvesting circuits

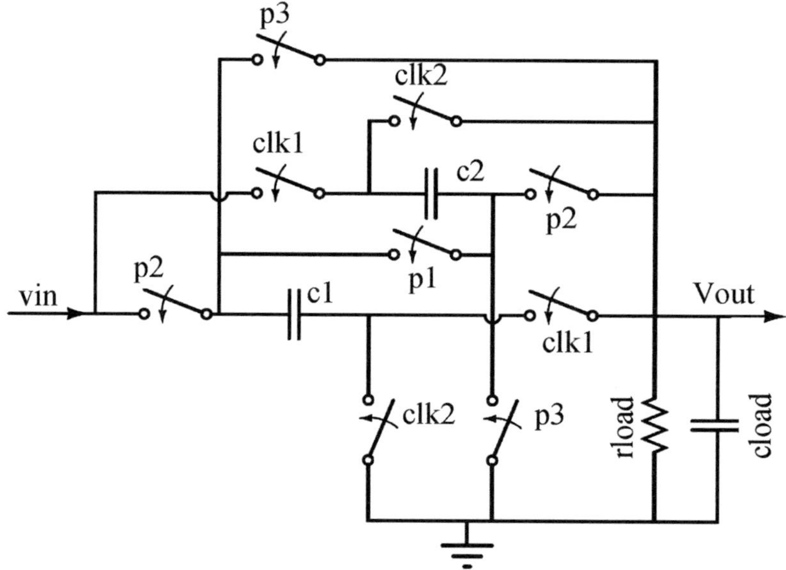

Fig. 5.26 Topology of the SC converter

ratio selector." The "Output voltage monitor" serves as a voltage detector by sending a signal to enable or disable the clock signal in order to confine the output voltage. The oscillator and the "Clock generator and controller" generate the non-overlapping clocks for the switched capacitor converter. The ultra-low voltage "LDO (Low Drop-Out) regulator with wide band PSR" supplies the regulated output voltage. The "Bandgap reference" provides the precise bias current and reference voltage for the LDO and switched capacitor converter. The control signals of the switched capacitor converter are generated by the "Step-down ratios selector."

Table 5.3 Step-down ratio vs. control signals A and B

Ratio	1/3	1/2	2/3
A	0	1	1
B	1	2	0

Table 5.4 PZT power harvesting circuit performance summary (simulated)

Symbol	Parameter	Value
V_{DD}	Supply voltage	1.5~2.1 V
V_{out}	Output voltage	0.3~0.6 V
I_{load}	Maximum load	0.8 mA
I_Q	Quiescent current	<150 μA
μ_{tot}	Power efficiency	66~74 %
T_R	Response time	<200 μs
V_{over}	Overshoot voltage	<5 mV
V_{pp}	Output voltage ripple	<1 mV

The topology of the switched capacitor converter is shown in Fig. 5.10, which is illustrated in detail in [23]. The control signals A and B are generated by the "Step-down ratios selector" and their values (shown in Table 5.3) are determined by the step-down ratio. A and B are used to select different step-down conversion ratios. p1, p2, and p3 are logic combinations of A, B, clk1 and clk2, respectively, as illustrated in Table 5.3. Equations (5.2), (5.3), and (5.4) show the relationship between p1, p2, p3, and other signals.

$$p1 = clk1 * A + clk2 * B \tag{5.2}$$

$$p2 = clk1 * A \tag{5.3}$$

$$p3 = clk2 * B \tag{5.4}$$

The ultra-low voltage LDO regulator with a wideband PSR is designed with the Feed Forward Ripple Cancellation (FFRC) technique [24]. The supply ripples generated by the switched capacitor converter, appearing at the source of the pass transistor, are reproduced on the gate of the pass transistor using the feed-forward path. Thus, the gate-source voltage of the pass transistor is free of ripples. The main advantage of this FFRC approach is achieving a high PSR for a wide frequency range without increasing the loop bandwidth. Such an approach significantly reduces quiescent power consumption [24]. Besides, this approach preserves the same LDO voltage of the conventional regulator, since PSR does not occur on the high-current signal path.

In the presented design, the minimum input of the LDO with the FFRC technique is 0.75 V and the output voltage ranges from 0.3 to 0.6 V. The lowest drop-out voltage is 0.15 V.

The performance of the PZT power harvesting circuit is shown in Table 5.4. The conversion efficiency of LDO can reach 82 %, and the efficiency of the whole harvesting system ranges from 66 to 74 % for a load current of 800 μA.

5.2 Low Power Digital Controller for SIDs

In an application system, the control unit (CU) can be implemented using either a general-purpose microcontroller (MCU) or a finite-state machine (FSM) logic circuit. From the view point of power consumption and power efficiency, the FSM would be better than MCU, as for the same control function, an FSM logic circuit consumes much less power than MCU, even those MCUs with the ultra-low-power mode. For those applications that need relatively complicated data processing, an FSM logic circuit can be fully optimized in terms of clock speed, power consumption, chip area, etc. For those applications that require very simple control flow, an MCU turns to be over-design. However, an MCU can provide the flexibility that an FSM logic circuit cannot have. For those applications that require very complicated control flows, an FSM logic circuit will need a large number of states or a multi-level state machine, which makes the design and verification quite complicated, and even imposes some potential risk when the state machine complexity increases. On the contrary, an MCU with certain programmability will make the control unit design flow quite simple, convenient, and robust.

The wireless medical and health care SIDs have some special concerns to design the digital control circuit which performs the system flow control and data processing. To achieve the highest reliability, these systems usually require a relatively complicated control flow to cover all the possible abnormities and emergencies. It will be difficult to implement such a flow controller using an FSM circuit. A programmable MCU will be quite suitable to accomplish this task. For the data processing part, such as the image data compression, it would not be a good choice to use the MCU program to do the computation, as the MCU would require a high speed system clock and therefore quite high power consumption to do the processing.

A nature solution is to combine a customized MCU and some application-oriented accelerators to implement the digital circuit for the SoCs used for wireless medical and health care SIDs. The customized MCU is in charge of the high-level system flow control, and the accelerators take the responsibility of data processing. This solution will give the system flexibility, reliability, and power efficiency simultaneously.

To illustrate the SID digital controller design methods, the SIDs can be divided into two categories with different purposes:

- "Sensing": these SIDs usually (continuously) collect body information. They perform the application procedure "sensing—processing—radio" during data/information gathering.
- "Intervention": these SIDs usually give bioelectrical pulse-intervention or perform drug-delivery. The preferred procedure is usually "radio—parsing—stimulating."

To achieve the best energy utilization from batteries, module-level co-operations of the entire SID must be optimized. All the sub-modules are controlled by the customized MCU, which schedules each task from both software level and hardware level. For example, according to the general control flow of SIDs, data path, and control path should be elaborated specifically to satisfy low-power and adequate performance.

For either purpose, energy consumed in the radio phase contributes the largest percentage in total energy consumption. To improve efficiency, it demands not only a low-power MCU core to perform good control flow and communication flow, but also a hardware medium access controller (MAC), which can accelerate link operations and reduce energy wastage (e.g., RF is on but no data to transmit) [25, 26].

Additionally, to improve performance of critical operations, modifications in instruction set (e.g., for DMA and I/Os) can bring benefits of code compression and accelerated execution. Also, mass data transferring will not need MCU to execute so many operations as previously. Instead, the MCU can stay in idle state while mass data accessing.

Remote reprogrammable feature is also practical and necessary for SIDs. Wireless field programming arbiter (WFPA) supports remotely online configuration, including SFRs and program memory. This provides much flexibility for the SIDs which need software (program) updating after being installed.

There are some additional requirements that the implementation contains multimode peripheral interface including I^2C, SPI, and general purpose parallel ports for I/O flexibility. The interrupt controller must be elaborated to ensure the robustness when exception occurs. Since security is not so strict in SIDs, we can implement simple security algorithm in MCU program.

Note that the MCU in the SoC requires almost no computation, so the customized MCU can be optimized to reduce the complexity and save power consumption.

5.2.1   SID Controller Design

This subsection will give the design details of an SID controller.

General Control Flows of SIDs

Generally, the sensing SIDs have different control flows from those intervention SIDs. Figure 5.27 shows control flows for both the sensing SIDs and intervention SIDs. For many cases, the half-duplex wireless channel is used for the data communication link [26, 27].

There are many kinds of sensor (or transducer) devices for SIDs. Because the schemes with multipurpose peripheral sensor interfaces are adopted in many researches, there appears almost no difference between control flows in SIDs with various sensors.

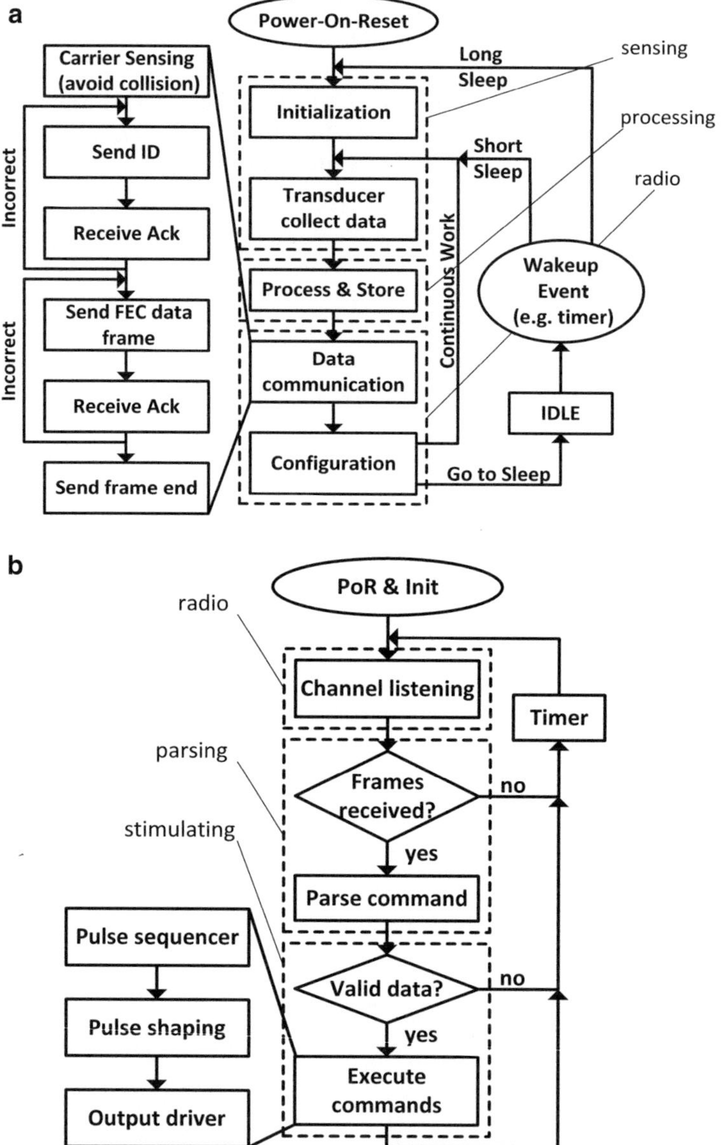

Fig. 5.27 Control flows of (**a**) sensing SIDs and (**b**) intervention SIDs

Sensing SIDs

The corresponding control flow for a sensing ID is shown in Fig. 5.27a. With the control flow, the SIDs can accomplish the sensing–processing–communicating–executing flow under supervision of the PBS. The remote PBS can also configure the SIDs' states and modes through this control flow.

The uplink (from SIDs to the PBS) is for biomedical information data transmission and the downlink (from the PBS to SIDs) is for configuration commands and acknowledgements (ACK). Forward error controlling (FEC) and automatic repeat request (ARQ) are utilized to ensure communication quality.

The sensing phase usually has a very little duty cycle to reduce energy consumption. In the processing phase, the SIDs probably calculate or directly store the data from the sensing phase, depending on the specific function. The radio phase establishes communication link and transmits/receives data in the storage.

In this control flow, SIDs can wake up when triggered by "wakeup" events: a local time-out signal from the timer, a remote signal from the PBS, etc.

Intervention SIDs

The corresponding control flow is shown in Fig. 5.27b. With this simplified control flow, the SIDs will be kept in the channel-listening state for most of the lifetime. Once a command frame received, SIDs come back to work, parse the command, and take actions if (and only if) it is valid.

In this scenario, the downlink is preferred and the uplink is rarely used. The SIDs can work either periodically or on-demand, based on the power-saving mode.

In the radio phase, SIDs receive commands from the PBS, parse the command frame to go through proper configurations, and then drive the corresponding output driver modules to make interventions.

Controller Design and Implementation

The proposed architecture of MCU is shown in Fig. 5.28. The entire controlled contains a basic 8051-compatible MCU core, MAC, WFPA, accelerator for preprocessing, DMA controller, memories, timers, multipurpose peripheral interface, debug interface, etc.

Optimizations

As mentioned above, the most important requirements of SIDs are low power, high efficiency, good flexibility, and robustness.

The sensing SIDs require periodical work mode, sparsely used downlink and busy uplink with relatively higher data rate. The intervention–function SIDs may require only downlink to receive appropriate parameters for the pulse stimulating or drug delivery actions. These unbalanced characteristics can be solved better using a customized MAC protocol [25, 27].

To achieve low power, the block-level and fine-grained gating techniques are extremely used to eliminate the excessive power of inactive modules and DFFs.

The acceleration instructions for memory access are added to the existing instructions set, making the program code more compact. The high-efficiency DMA

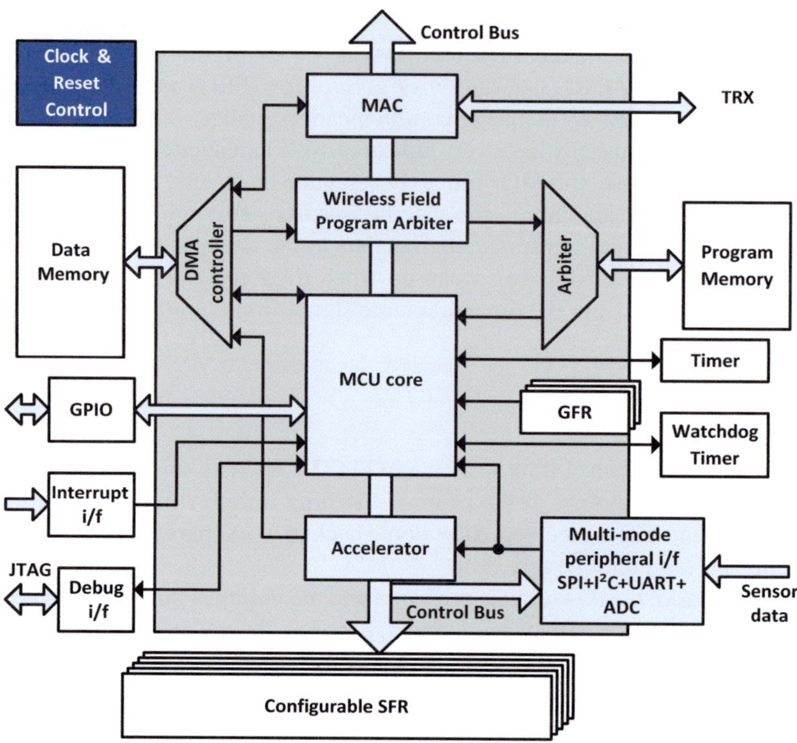

Fig. 5.28 SID digital controller architecture

controller also improves the system energy efficiency, especially for the situations of mass data transferring and processing. Additionally, hardware MAC integrates channel encoding/decoding, scramble, CDR, and frame control.

With the WFPA, the SIDs can be reprogrammed remotely by the BS whenever needed, which brings in great convenience and flexibility. Moreover, the multipurpose peripheral interface supports universal synchronous/asynchronous receiver/transmitter (USART), such as SPI, I²C, and RS-232 [28, 29].

MCU Core

The MCU core has a basic 8051-compatible instruction set, which is adequate to implement star-topology single-hop network protocols suitable for SIDs. So a common non-pipelined Harvard architecture is adopted in the MCU.

For typical SID functions, the memory operations take up to over 40 % of the entire operations. The most frequent section appears like:

```
...
for (addr=0; addr<tnum; addr++)
{   tbuf = datamem[offset+addr];
```

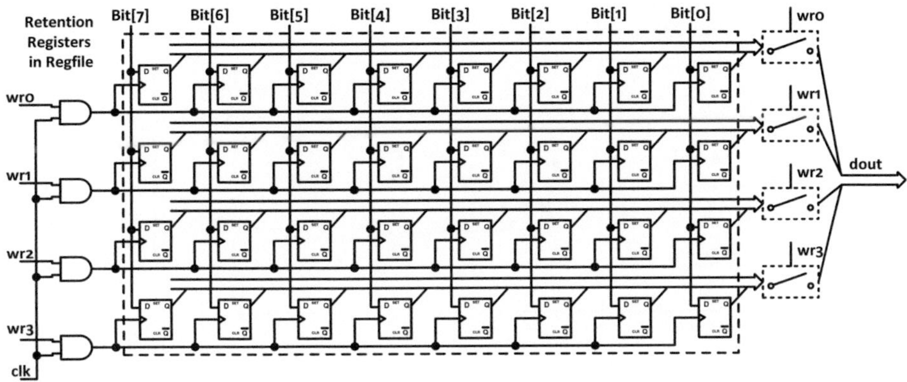

Fig. 5.29 Schematic of retention registers

```
while (TBUF_ALMOST_FULL);
  }
  ...
```

After compilation, the assemble codes take about 20 instructions (or even more). Furthermore, the corresponding binary codes may execute $20*t_{num}$ operations according to the section, approximately.

Several accelerating instructions are added to the instruction set, which can improve code length and execution efficiency. As a result, the $20*t_{num}$ operations (imply equal quantity of memory accesses) can be reduced to only three operations:

```
...
MOV DMADDR, offset
MOV DMANUM, tnum
DMAOP
...
```

These optimizations in instruction set can bring in high efficiency.

Retention registers are also necessary to hold values and states when the MCU is powered off (in the max power-saving modes of SIDs). These registers are powered directly by the battery; while other modules of MCU are all powered by a DC-DC power supply. Figure 5.29 shows the schematic of a typical kind of retention registers.

Medium Access Controller

Based on the above analysis, both sensing and intervention functions are considered. The MAC module consists of two separate controllers for transmitting and receiving, as shown in Fig. 5.30.

The TX path achieves data framing and streaming, including channel coding such as CRC, Reed-Solomon encoding, and whitening. The TX controller sets/resets the logic modules and enables/disables the RF front end modules.

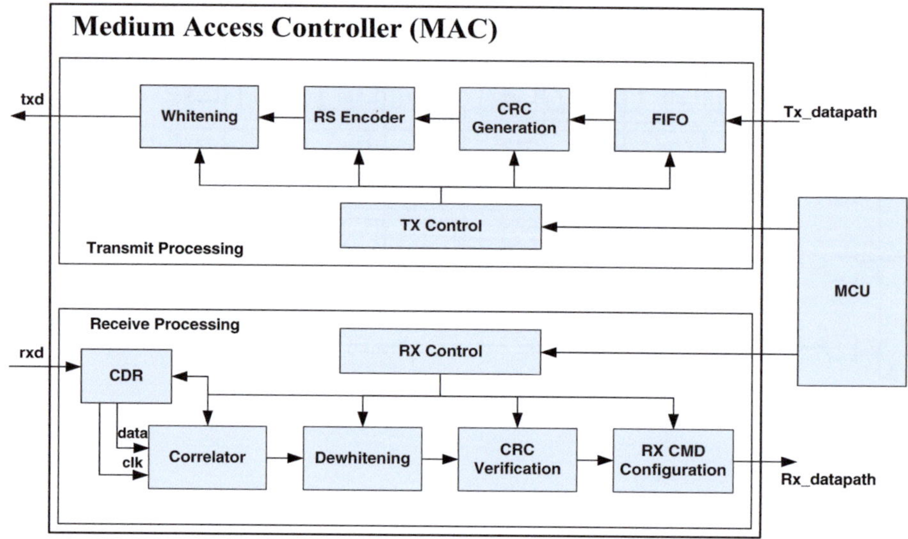

Fig. 5.30 Block Diagram of MAC

CRC-24 is adopted, and the corresponding polynomial is:

$$x^{24}+x^{23}+x^{18}+x^{17}+x^{14}+x^{11}+x^{10}+x^7+x^6+x^5+x^4+x^3+x+1.$$

RS(31, 25) coding scheme is utilized, of which there are 5 bits per symbol and the primitive polynomial is x^5+x^2+1.

Scrambles (whitening) are useful to avoid consecutive 0s and 1s. A three-order polynomial of x^3+x^2+1 is adequate for common purpose.

The RX path achieves CDR firstly, and then makes decisions for bit synchronous and frame synchronous. De-whitening and CRC modules are corresponding to the TX path. For the SIDs, the RX link is quite different from the TX link: RX does not need high speed and mass data, so that there is no need to use RS coding in the link and RS decoder does not appear in the Rx path.

WFPA and DMA Controller

Remotely reprogrammable feature is supported by the WFPA module. It is very practical and necessary for SIDs because: once the SID is installed inside the body, it will be very hard (or impossible) to take outside again even if there is a need to update the software. WFPA supports remotely online configuration and software update, suitable for rewriting both program memory (E^2PROM, FLASH, etc.) and specific function registers (SFRs).

DMA controller accomplishes mass data accessing as:

- Tx data path for data communication, from data memory to RF MAC.
- Rx data path for command communication, from RF MAC to data memory.
- WFPA data path, from data memory to instruction memory.

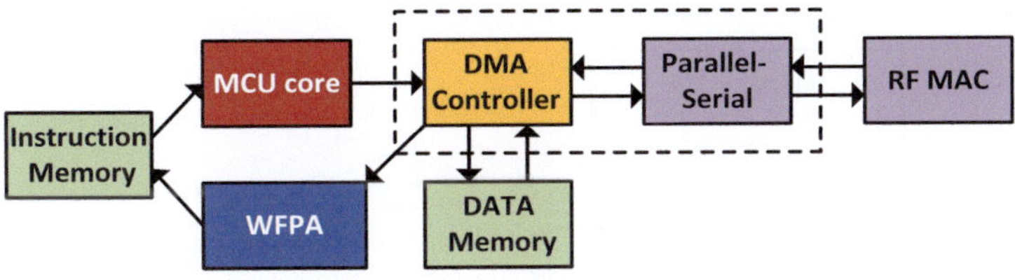

Fig. 5.31 Data path with WFPA and DMAC

The data path is shown in Fig. 5.31. Program code for remote updating should be stored in data memory during previous communication. Once the DMA controller assigns corresponding channel for WFPA, WFPA can overwrite the instruction memory all through from the data memory. Every time the MCU wakes up and back to work, its key status must be restored and guaranteed by CRC-8 verification.

Implementation Results

The proposed SID digital controller has been fabricated in standard 0.18 μm CMOS technology, occupying 1.4×0.8 mm die area, with 79.1 K equivalent gates and 6.6 kB on-chip memory (2.6 kB for program and 4 kB for data).

When powered by 1.8 V DC-DC supply, the controller consumes 510 μA under the condition of 13 MHz clock, 2.5 Mbps avg. throughput, with a program code of 1:8 duty-cycle for the application case of body temperature sensing. When powered by 0.9 V power supply, the power consumption is only 165 μW. Its power consumption can be even lowered to 42 μW under operation-idle conditions. The peripheral sensor device and the RF module for verification are proved correctly behavior.

In summary, a low-power, energy-efficient digital controller using a customized MCU has been designed, with the remotely programmable feature. Both for sensing and intervention SIDs, the presented controller can help to achieve concise program code and energy efficient operations, based on the improved MCU core instruction set and the DMA channels. The controller also provides good flexibility for SIDs to be compatible with common I/O bus interfaces and to be able to update software remotely by the PBS. The prototype has been verified using an FPGA board, and fabricated and validated on silicon.

5.2.2   Subthreshold MCU

In order to further save SID power consumption, a subthreshold MCU can be used to replace the MCU using standard working voltages. The architecture of the 8-bit MCU is plotted in Fig. 5.32. The "Internal ROM" which contains a 128-byte SRAM is programmed to test the system functions. The "Control unit" (CU) is the control center of the MCU. The Arithmetic Logic Unit (ALU), the Operation-Program Decoder

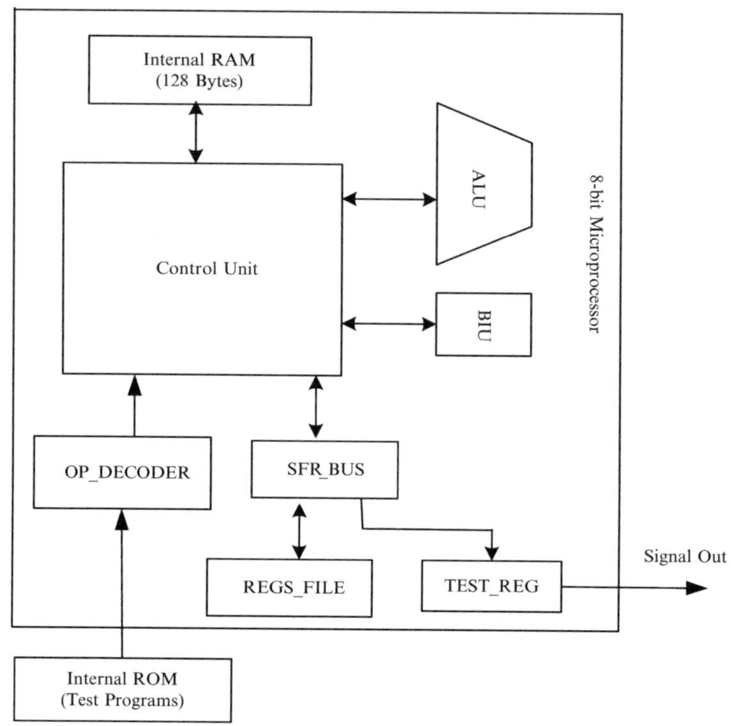

Fig. 5.32 Architecture of the subthreshold MCU

Table 5.5 Simulation comparisons between 32-bit subthreshold and standard CLAs

Synthesized library	Frequency (KHz)	Leakage (nA)	Dynamic (nW)	PDP (pJ)	EDP (pJ·µs)	Cell amount
Subthreshold	690	2	45	0.07	0.08	343
Standard	501	5	90	0.18	0.36	349
Comparison	37 %↑	60 %↓	50 %↓	61 %	77 %	≈

(OP_DECODER), the Register file (REGS_FILE), and the Bus Interface Unit (BIU) are also designed for the MCU. An 8-bit Testing Register (TEST_REG) is added to the internal Special Function Register Bus (SFR_BUS). The output signal can be detected by an oscilloscope. The MCU is fully compatible with the 8051 MCU.

The standard inverter is sized to achieve low leakage and maximal noise margin that is very important for subthreshold circuit. The subthreshold library in the design contains about 80 cells which can be designed with the standard CAD tools and design flow.

A 32-bit Carry-Look-ahead-Adder (CLA) is simulated for evaluation. The measurements results of the longest path for average frequency, the power-including leakage and dynamic as well as the Power-Delay Product (PDP) and Energy-Delay Product (EDP) are listed in Table 5.5. For comparison, the adders are synthesized

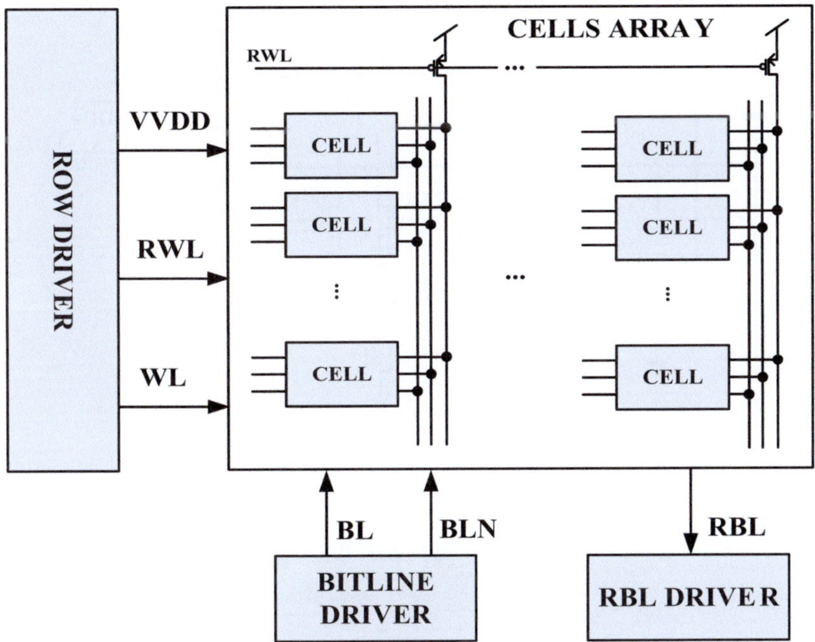

Fig. 5.33 SRAM structure

with conventional 180 nm standard library and subthreshold library, respectively. Judging from the results, all the performances of the subthreshold adder are much better than that with the standard library.

The structure of the RAM is depicted in Fig. 5.33. The drivers along with the address decoders including the "ROW DRIVER," the "BITLINE DRIVER" and the "RBL DRIVER" are synthesized by the combinational logic for stability. The "Cell Array" is designed with the improved 11-T subthreshold cell (seen in Fig. 5.34). The 11-T subthreshold SRAM cell is constructed by a standard 6-T cell and a read-out-buffer (M_{7-11}).

The RBL (Read Bit Line) is connected to VDD during the idle time. That is different from that in the traditional design. As a result, it will increase the leakage current from VDD to GND through the read-out buffer when all cells saves "0". To mitigate the problem, an extra transistor (M_{11} in Fig. 5.34) is added to the cell. When the RBL is connected to VDD, all cells *save* "1" to the RBL to suppress the leakage. It means that more cells can be connected to the RBL theoretically. There are three main advantages:

1. The conventional pre-charge process of RBL is bypassed to accelerate the speed.
2. The system stability is enhanced. In the ultra-low voltage domain, the float RBL will be easily disturbed by parasitic capacitance due to the random noise.
3. The speed is accelerated. For the delay time of reading logic "1" is zero, the delay time depends only on the current discharge time through the NMOS stack. In this technology, NMOS is much stronger than PMOS (about ten times).

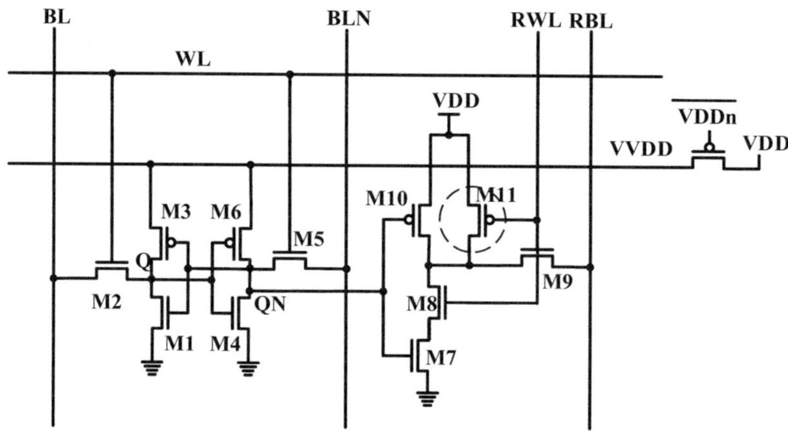

Fig. 5.34 11-T SRAM cell structure

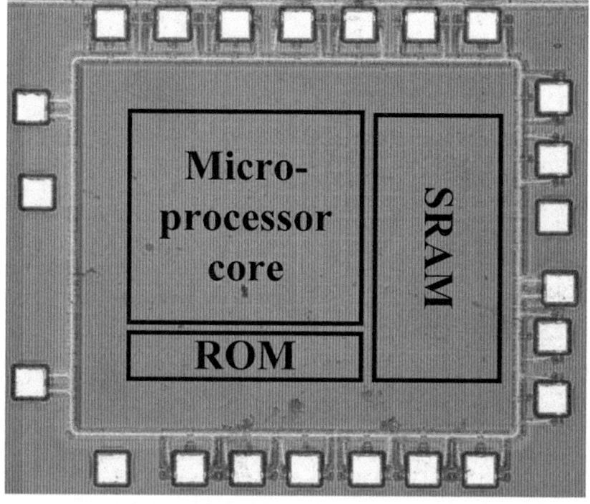

Fig. 5.35 Subthreshold MCU micrograph

The MCU was fabricated in 0.18 μm CMOS process for demonstration. The die size is 1.3*1 mm shown in Fig. 5.35. The performance summary of the MCU is listed in Table 5.6.

From Table 5.6, it can be seen that the leakage power of the MCU is only 46 nW and the dynamic power 385nW@165 kHz with the operating voltage of 350 mV. The energy per instruction is about 13 pJ.

Besides, the measurement results also show that the subthreshold MCU can operate with a supply voltage as low as 250 mV except the operations of the memory. With the supply voltage of 350 mV, the MCU can operate at a rate of up to 1.5 MHz.

Table 5.6 Performance summary of the subthreshold MCU

VDD (V)	Leakage (nW)	Dynamic (µW)	Frequency (MHz)	Energy/inst (pJ/inst)
0.35	46	0.385	0.16	13
0.4	56	1.52	0.33	18.8
0.45	65	5.13	0.8	13.3
0.5	75	15	1.9	25.2
0.6	120	61.8	5.5	23.2
0.7	180	143.5	11	27.5

5.2.3   Accelerator Design Example: A JPEG-LS Compressor

As mentioned above, for a specific SID, application-oriented accelerators can be implemented for complicated data processing, as the MCU core does not have the computation ability. This subsection will show the design details of a JPEG-LS image compression accelerator which can be used for the capsule endoscope SID.

The image compression accelerator is dedicatedly designed for a CMOS image sensor with Bayer color filter array (CFA). For image data in the CFA format, there is only one color component in each pixel and the other two color components for the given pixel need to be interpolated using neighboring pixel information to generate a full color image. In most applications, the full color image is compressed before storage or transmission which results in three times data amount and processing time compared to the CFA image. The method proposed in [30] avoids this data redundancy by moving the compression stage before color interpolation. By compressing the CFA pattern before the interpolation, more pertinent information is retained, allowing a higher compression rate while maintaining the image quality [31]. Furthermore, this scheme could greatly save the hardware cost such as the on-chip memory storage and the communication bandwidth for wireless data transmission. For these reasons, the Bayer CFA pattern is directly compressed and transmitted in the proposed image compression module. The VLSI architecture of the image compression module is shown in Fig. 5.36. It is composed of an image filter and a JPEG-LS encoder which will be described in detail next.

Hardware-Oriented Image Filter

A characteristic associated with the Bayer CFA pattern is that for a given pixel the neighboring pixels always belong to different color components, as shown in Fig. 5.37. The correlation between two neighboring pixels is very low and the influence of high spatial frequencies is extremely notable. Therefore, algorithms based on prediction such as DPCM, or based on transformation such as DWT, suffer from a severe degradation on the compression performance. In this work, an image filter algorithm is introduced to alleviate this problem.

Several filter algorithms have been proposed in [32, 33], which improve the performance of JPEG-LS notably while still maintaining the reconstructed images' quality high.

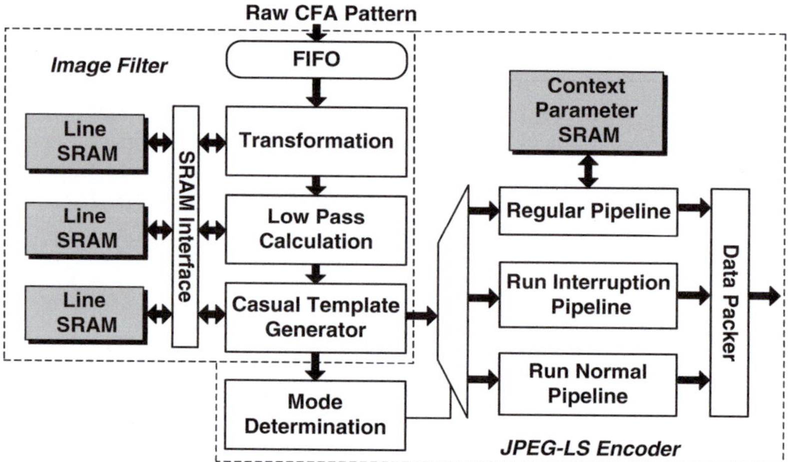

Fig. 5.36 Block diagram of the JPEG-LS image compression module

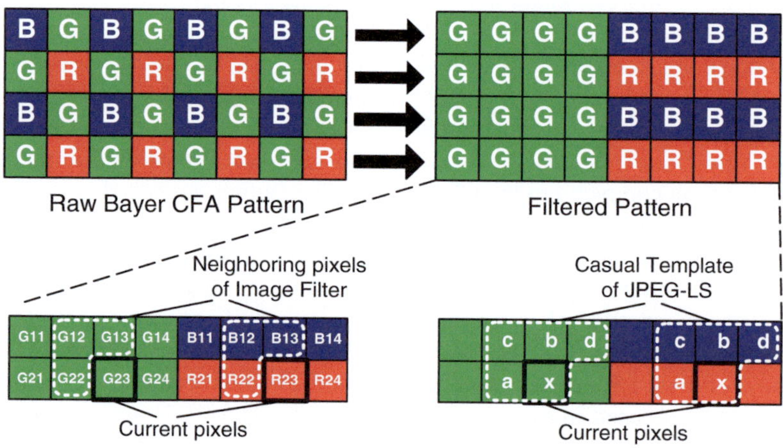

Fig. 5.37 Proposed image filtering process and casual template generation of JPEG-LS algorithm

However, these methods are not hardware-oriented. In these methods, the B, G, and R components are preprocessed and compressed individually, but the JPEG-LS encoder can handle only one component at a time. So the other two components have to wait for their turns, which cause large storage consumption as well as long processing time. For the purpose of real-time data processing and low memory requirement, a real-time image filter algorithm has been proposed, in which the data are firstly transformed and then low-pass filtered directly in RGB space to depress the high spatial frequencies. Afterwards, the casual template is generated and sent to the JPEG-LS encoder for compression, as shown in Fig. 5.36. The decompressed data can be reconstructed by reversing the process. As illustrated in Fig. 5.37, the G component and the B and R components are separated into two rectangular arrays by transformation operation. The high spatial frequencies between neighboring pixels due to different color component belonging are greatly decreased, which helps the following JPEG-LS encoder helpful to obtain a relative high compression rate for. In the presented method, B and R components are processed together as a single color component in the filtering procedure. As a contrary, if all the three color components are treated individually as what have been done in [33], a higher compression ratio would be obtained since the contexts modeling of JPEG-LS would be more precise, and the context of B, G, and R would not interact with each other. However, to process the three components individually will require a large amount of on-chip storage and large power consumption, not mentioning the inevitably increased processing time. These disadvantages are unacceptable for a high performance VLSI implementation. To make a good compromise between the cost and the performance, two-color-components filter method is used in this design as described above. The filtering algorithm can be implemented in two steps.

[**Step 1**]. *Transformation: G components and B and R components are separated into two rectangular arrays.*

$$\begin{cases} X = x \\ Y = y + \left(\left(-1 \right)^{x+y} + 1 \right) \cdot N / 4 \end{cases} \tag{5.5}$$

where (x, y) is the coordination of the current pixel, while (X, Y) indicates the coordination after transformation. N indicates the width of the image.
[**Step 2**]. *Low pass filtering: the current pixel is averaged with the neighboring pixels within both horizontal and vertical direction.*

$$P'_{(X,Y)} = \frac{1}{4} \left(\left(P_{(X,Y)} + P'_{(X-1,Y-1)} + 1 \right) + \left(P'_{(X-1,Y)} + P'_{(X,Y-1)} + 1 \right) \right) \tag{5.6}$$

where P indicates the original value of the current pixel, P' indicates the filtered value.

For the current pixel, the filtering algorithm only utilizes the available past neighboring pixels within casual template of the JPEG-LS algorithm. By doing so, it helps to achieve real-time operation with small memory storage, and also facilitates the causal template generation of JPEG-LS. Due to the limited bit width, the division operation in (5.5) will introduce error that no more than two after reconstruction.

In order to evaluate the compression performance, the proposed algorithm is compared to the standard JPEG-LS (without the image filter) and the method proposed in [33]. The CFA raw data for evaluation are generated from several standard color images with VGA resolution. Compared to the standard JPEG-LS, the method with image filtering has better image quality and higher compression rate, and would be a better choice in consideration of the hardware overhead, storage cost, and the overall processing time.

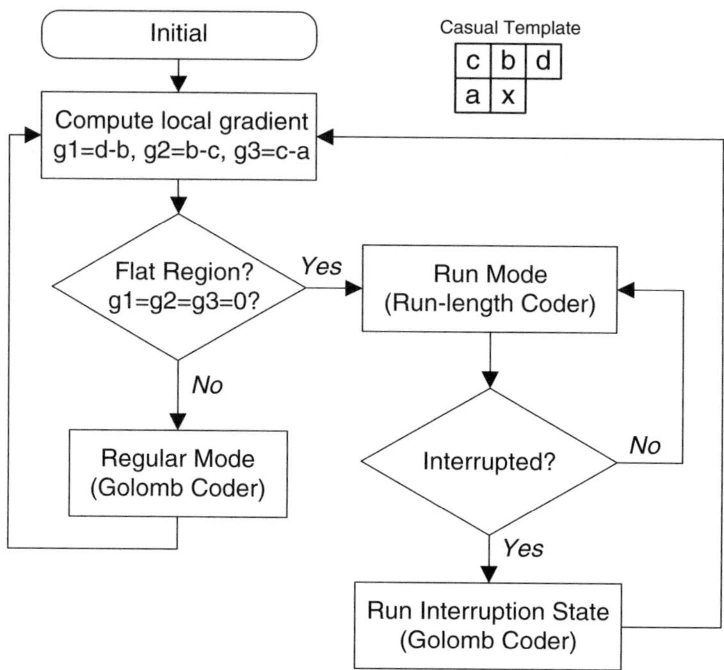

Fig. 5.38 Simplified flow diagram of JPEG-LS algorithm

JPEG-LS Encoder

JPEG-LS is an established standard for lossless and near-lossless compression of still images [34]. It provides both the highest lossless compression ratio and the fastest compression speed for medical images. The main compression techniques of JPEG-LS [35] can be summarized as follows:

- *Context modeling*: It performs local gradient computation, gradient quantization, and quantized gradient merging.
- *Context-based statistic*: Context parameters A[Q], B[Q], C[Q], and N[Q] are iterated for each context model.
- *Predictor*: It is composed of fixed predictor and adaptive correction. The prediction residual is calculated for coding.
- *Run-length coding*: It is used for the smooth local region.
- *Limited-length Golomb coding*: It is used for prediction residual coding.

Figure 5.38 shows the simplified flow chart, in which a simple mode selection strategy is adopted. Based on the local gradient (g1, g2, g3) computation, each pixel would be encoded either in the regular mode or in the run mode by Golomb coder or run-length coder. The computation in the regular mode and the run interruption state contributes the most to the computation complexity of the JPEG-LS algorithm. The mapped prediction residual computation in the regular mode is always the most time-consuming part. Moreover, the update of context parameters A[Q], B[Q], C[Q], and N[Q] requires extra accessing time of memory. Thus, appropriate hardware architecture has to be considered to meet the real-time processing requirement. Several researches have explored such kind of hardware architecture. In [36], a limited parallelism is obtained only when the computation does not depend on the previous context history. In [37, 38], large on-chip memory and logic gates are sacrificed to exchange for higher throughput. However, none of these three methods can realize the real-time processing. The design in [39] implements efficient pipeline architecture with real-time processing capability. However, in the method proposed in [39], the parameter C[Q] is accessed concurrently by different pipeline stages, which requires double-sized context memory and inevitably increases the chip area.

To achieve an area and power efficient VLSI implementation of the JPEG-LS encoder, the proposed data path is optimized targeting the minimum resource utilization and power consumption. In this design, three parallel three-stage pipelined data paths are implemented. The three pipelines take care of the regular mode, the run mode and the run interruption state, respectively, as shown in Fig. 5.39. Only one of the three pipelines is activated according to the mode determination, which avoids the unnecessary computation of the other two pipelines for each pixel. Simulation shows that separated pipelines for different modes would result in an average of 90 % power reduction in the run mode. This is expected when considering the low computation complexity of the run pipeline. With this method, unnecessary switch activities are effectively reduced, especially when images are smooth. In addition, resource sharing is used among pipelines for common computation such as Golomb parameter k computation in the second stage and Golomb coder in the third stage, as shown in the dark gray color in Fig. 5.39.

For each pipeline stage, four clock processing cycles are allocated. This may degrade the throughput of the JPEG-LS encoder a little bit. However, this does not matter since in the endoscope system the wireless transmission presents a bottleneck, and a JPEG-LS encoder with very high throughput is not necessary for this application. Moreover, four clock processing cycles for each stage provide several advantages for a power and area efficient implementation. First, the in-stage resource sharing can be widely used to reduce the gate counts. Secondly, neither double-sized context memory nor dual port memory is required since the access of context memory can be finished in a single pipeline stage.

A two-level hierarchy memory access method is proposed to eliminate unnecessary memory accesses in the process of context parameters updating. For 365 quantized context models, four context parameters A[Q](14 bits), B[Q](6 bits), C[Q](8 bits), and N[Q](6 bits) have to be accumulated. A $34bits \times 365words$ single port SRAM is used for this purpose. Normally, for each pixel with a specific context, the four parameters would be read out and written back to SRAM in a specific address. However, these extensive memory accesses would consume considerable energy. The key observation is that the neighboring pixels from image filter have a great probability to own the same quantized context model due to the transformation in image filter, which means that the same address of context memory will be accessed continuously, though unnecessarily. To reduce the context memory accesses, the context parameters are first cached in registers in the third stage of the regular pipeline. The context memory would be accessed only if the next pixel encounters a different context

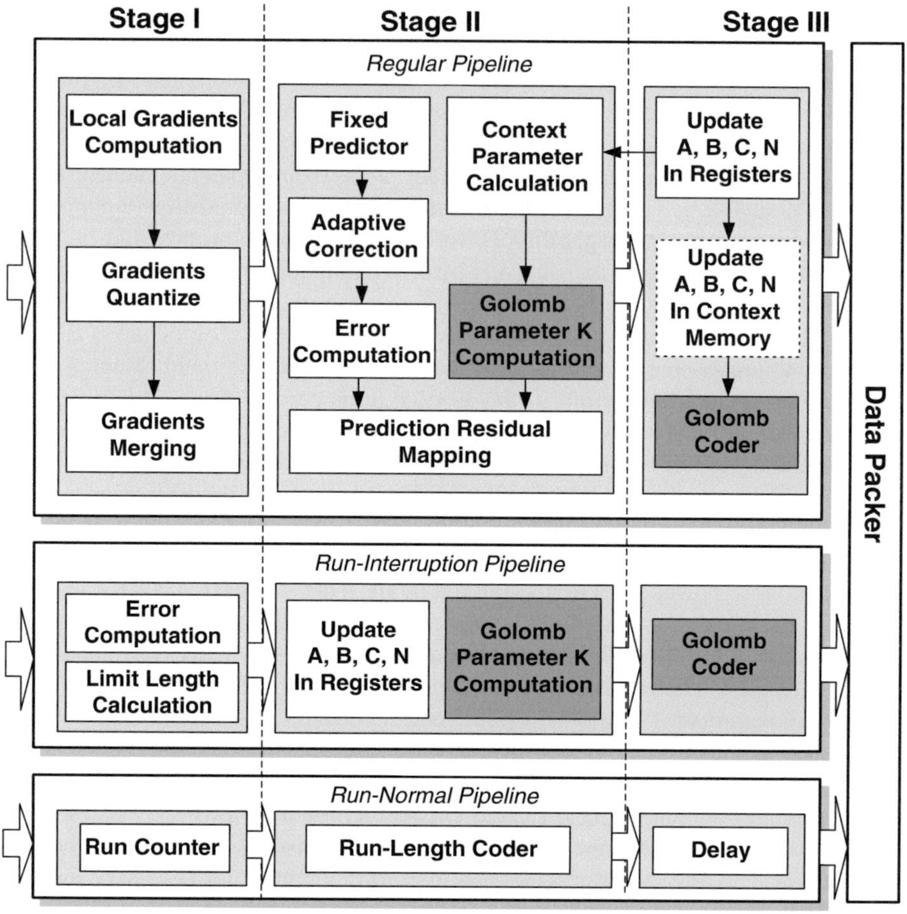

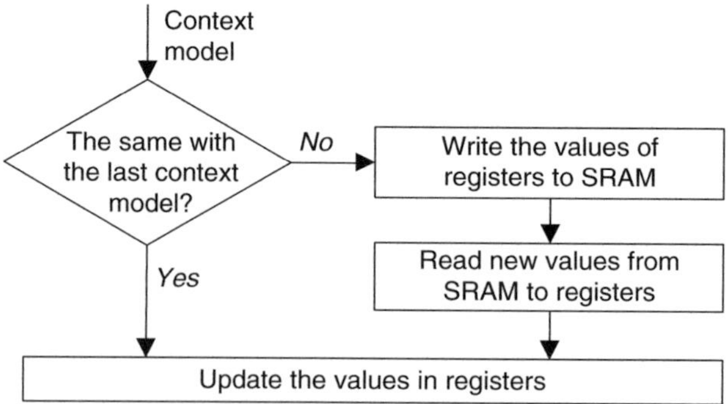

Fig. 5.39 Data path of JPEG-LS with three pipelines

Fig. 5.40 Hierarchy memory access method

model; otherwise, the value of registers would be used for accumulation without memory access, as shown in Fig.5.40. The experiments have shown that the proposed method results in an average of 52 % context memory accesses reduction which means considerable power reduction.

References

1. Sun T, Xie X, Wang Z. Wireless power transfer for medical microsystems. New York: Springer; 2013.
2. Renata 380 battery technical data sheet, available online at www.renata.com
3. Hammes M, Kranz C, Seippel D, et al. Evolution on SoC integration: GSM baseband-radio in 0.13μm CMOS extended by fully integrated power management unit. IEEE J Solid-State Circuits. 2008;43(1):236–44.
4. Rincon-Mora GA, Allen PE. A low-voltage, low quiescent current, low drop-out regulator. IEEE J Solid-State Circuits. 1998;33(1):36–44.
5. Fiocchi CG. A very flexible BiCMOS low-voltage high- performance source follower. ISCAS '99. 1999;2:212–5.
6. Ahuja BK. An improved frequency compensation technique for CMOS operational amplifiers. IEEE J Solid-State Circuits. 1983;18(6):629–33.
7. Iddan G, Meron G, Glukhovsky A, Swain P. Wireless capsule endoscopy. Nature. 2000;405:417.
8. Ginsberg GG, Barkun AN, Bosco JJ, Isenberg GA, Nguyen CC, Petersen BT, Silverman WB, Slivka A, Taitelbaum G. Wireless capsule endoscopy. Gastrointest Endosc. 2002;56(5): 621–4.
9. Dickson JF. On-chip high-voltage generation in MNOS integrated circuits using an improved voltage multiplier technique. IEEE J Solid-State Circuits. 1976;11(3):374–8.
10. Karthaus U, Fischer M. Fully integrated passive UHF RFID transponder IC with 16.7-μW minimum RF input power. IEEE J Solid-State Circuits. 2003;38(10):1602–8.
11. Milanovic V, Gaitan M, Marshall JC, Zaghloul ME. CMOS foundry implementation of Schottky diodes for RF detection. IEEE Trans Electron Dev. 1996;43(12):2210–4.
12. Roundy S, Wright PK, Rabaey J. A study of low level vibrations as a power source for wireless sensor nodes. Comput Commun. 2003;26(11):1131–44.
13. Platt SR, Farritor S, Garvin K, Haider H. The use of piezoelectric ceramics for electric power generation within orthopedic implants. IEEE/ASME Trans Mech. 2005;10(4):455–61.
14. Shenck NS, Paradiso JA. Energy scavenging with shoe-mounted piezoelectrics. IEEE Micro. 2001;21(3):30–42.
15. Edmison J, Jones M, Nakad Z. Using piezoelectric materials for wearable electronic textiles. In: Proceedings of the 6th International Symposium on Wearable Computers (ISWC.02); 2002. p. 41–8.
16. Ottman GK, Hofmann HF, Lesieutre GA. Optimized piezoelectric energy harvesting circuit using step-down converter in discontinuous conduction mode. IEEE Trans Power Electron. 2003;18(2):696–703.
17. Roundy S. "The power of good vibrations", Lab Notes-Research from the College of Engineering, NW Hagood IV, "Development of micro-hydraulic transducer technology." In: Proceedings of the 10th International Conference. Adaptive Structures and Technologies. Paris, France; 1999. p. 71–81.
18. Engel TG. Energy conversion and high power pulse production using miniature piezoelectric compressors. IEEE Trans Plasma Sci. 2000;28(5):1338–40.
19. Taylor GW, Burns JR, Kammann SM, Powers WB, Welsh TR. The energy harvesting eel: a small subsurface ocean/river power generator. IEEE J Ocean Eng. 2001;26(4):539–47.
20. Stephen RP. Electric power generation within orthopaedic implants using piezoelectric ceramics. Thesis. University of Lincoln; 2000.

21. Hao W, Jia C, Chen H, Zhang C, Wang Z. Variable ratio step-down switched capacitor DC-DC converter in WMSoOI. J Semiconducotors. 2009;30(12):125008(1-5).
22. Piezo systems, INC., piezo stacks [Online]. http://www.piezo.com/prodstacks1.html
23. Makowski MS, Maksimovic D. ''. PESC'95 Record, 26th Annual IEEE(2). Atlanta, Georgia; 1995. p. 1215–21.
24. El-Nozahi M, Amer A, Torres J, et al. A 25mA 0.13μm CMOS LDO regulator with power-supply rejection better than −56dB up to 10MHz using a feedforward ripple-cancellation technique. IEEE Solid-State Circuits Conference (ISSCC'2009). San Francisco, CA; 2009. p. 330–32.
25. Demirko I, et al. MAC protocols for wireless sensor networks: a survey. IEEE Commun Mag. 2006;44(4):115–21.
26. Yoo J, et al. A 5.2mW Self-configured wearable body sensor network controller and a 12μW 54.9% efficieny wirelessly powered sensor for continuous health monitoring system. ISSCC Dig. Tech. Papers; 2009. p. 290–1.
27. Ye W, Heidemann J, Estrin D. An energy-efficient MAC protocol for wireless sensor networks. In: Proceedings of the IEEE 21th Annual Joint Conference of the IEEE Computer and Communications Societies. 2002;3:1567–76.
28. Puers R, Wouters P. Adaptive interface circuits for flexible monitoring of temperature and movement. Analog Integr Circuits Signal Process. 1997;14:193–206.
29. Yazdi N, Mason A, et al. A generic interface chip for capacitive sensors in low-power multi-parameter microsystems. Sens Actuators A. 2000;84:351–61.
30. Lee SY, Ortega A. A novel approach of image compression in digital cameras with a Bayer color filter array. IEEE Int Conf Image Process. 2001;3:482–5.
31. Koh CC, Mukherjee J, Mitra SK. New efficient methods of image compression in digital cameras with color filter array. IEEE Trans Consum Electron. 2003;49(4):1448–56.
32. Xie X, Li G, Li X. A new approach for near-lossless and lossless image compression with Bayer color filter arrays. ICIG 2004; Hong Kong. p. 357–60.
33. Xie X, Li G, Wang Z. A low complexity and high quality image compression method for digital cameras. ETRI Journal. 2006;28(2):260–3.
34. International Telecommunication Union. ITU-T Recommendation T.87. Information technology-lossless and near-lossless compression of continuous-tone images-baseline. https://www.itu.int/rec/dologin_pub.asp?lang=e&id=T-REC-T.87-199806-I!!ZPF-E&type=items, 1998.
35. Weinberger M, Seroussi G, Sapiro G. The LOCO-I lossless image compression algorithm: principles and standardization into JPEG-LS. IEEE Trans Image Process. 2000;9(8):1309–24.
36. Lee SY, Ortega A. A novel approach of image compression in digital cameras with a Bayer color filter array. In: Proceedings of the IEEE International Conference Image Process. 2001;3:482–5.
37. Savakis A, Pioriun M. Benchmarking and hardware implementation of JPEG-LS. ICIP'02. Rochester, NY. 2002.
38. Xie X, Li G, Chen X, Li X, Wang Z. A low-power digital IC design inside the wireless endo-scopic capsule. IEEE J Solid-State Circuits. 2006;41(11):2390–400.
39. Papadonikolakis M, Pantazis V, Kakarountas AP. Efficient high-performance ASIC implementation of JPEG-LS encoder. Design, Automation & Test in Europe Conference & Exhibition. 2007:1–6.

Chapter 6
SoC Design and Application Systems

6.1 Wireless Capsule Endoscope SoC and Application System

6.1.1 Wireless Capsule Endoscope SoC

According to the system requirement [1–4], the targeted SoC mainly performs the function of image data acquisition, processing, and transmission. The electrical part of a wireless capsule endoscope (WCE) with bidirectional communication can be built using this SoC and a CMOS image sensor. The major function blocks of this SoC include the digital controller, the RF wireless transceiver, the image data processing block, and the power management unit, as shown in Fig. 6.1. To meet the system requirement, the SoC should have the features of high integration level, low power consumption, and requiring very few external components.

The WCE SoC has an ultra-low-power (ULP) digital controller with a customized MCU for the flow control. The JPEG-LS image data compressor as presented in Chap. 5 is implemented as a hard accelerator to carry out lossless/near-lossless image compression. Such a compressor can achieve a compression ratio of ~1/3 [5, 6], which can greatly improve the system power efficiency.

The SoC has a half-duplex transceiver with asymmetric data rates for the transmitter and the receiver, which was introduced in Chap. 4. The transceiver works in the frequency range of 404–432 MHz which is divided into eight programmable frequency channels with 4 MHz intervals. The transmitter adopts an MSK modulation with 1/2/3 Mbps data rate, and the highest effective data transmission rate is about 2 Mbps. The receiver has an OOK demodulator, the highest receiving data rate is 64 kbps.

The SoC has three integrated linear low-dropout (LDO) regulators and one switched-capacitor boost regulator to provide supplies to the on-chip function blocks, the external image sensor, and the strobe light LEDs. The regulators are all programmable and the WCE power consumption can be optimized with appropriate voltage settings.

Z. Wang et al., *CMOS IC Design for Wireless Medical and Health Care,*
DOI 10.1007/978-1-4614-9503-1_6, © Springer Science+Business Media New York 2014

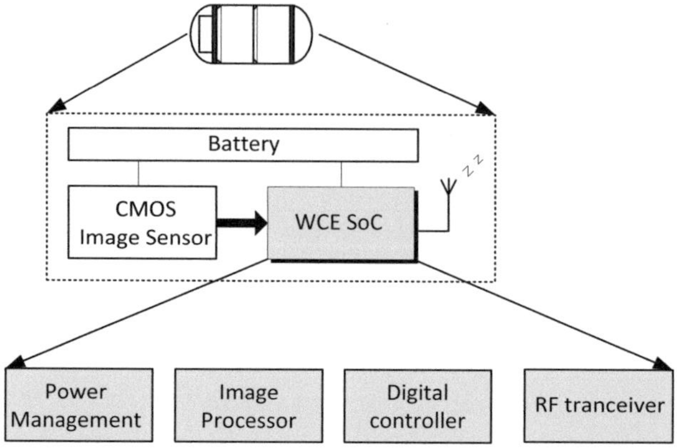

Fig. 6.1 Targeted SoC in a wireless capsule endoscope

WCE SoC Design Specifications

To fulfill the application requirement, the targeted WCE SoC should achieve the following design specifications.

1. Half-duplex bidirectional wireless communication

   - Eight programmable carrier frequencies: 404 MHz, 408 MHz, …, 432 MHz with 4 MHz intervals
   - Transmitter data rate up to 3 Mbps ([4] has a 2.7 Mbps transmitter) with the effective data rate up to 2 Mbps
   - Transmitter output power level ≥-20 dBm
   - Receiver sensitivity -85 dBm @ 10^{-3} raw bit-error-rate (BER) with 64 kbps data rate

2. Current consumption from 3 V power supply

   - ≤ 1 mA during image data acquisition and compression
   - ≤ 3 mA when transmitting image data
   - ≤ 8 mA when receiving commands from PBS
   - Standby current ≤ 200 μA
   - Leakage current ≤ 3 μA when powered down

3. Image data acquisition

   - Image data format: Raw Bayer
   - Image resolution: $480 \times 480 / 240 \times 240$

SoC Architecture

Based on the function requirement analysis, the target WCE SoC should have the following function blocks, as shown in Fig. 6.2.

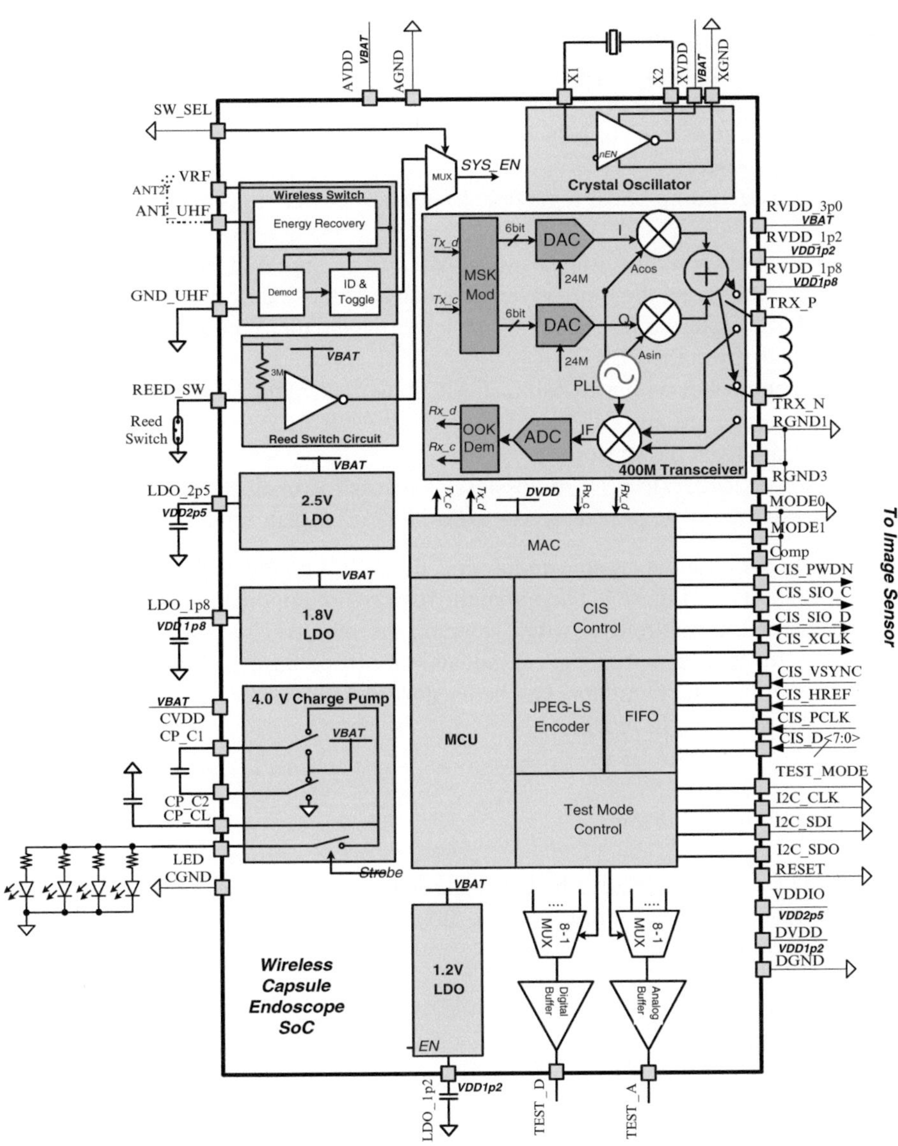

Fig. 6.2 WCE SoC function block diagram

- Wireless power switch: to provide the wireless access to the system power on/off
- Dry reed switch circuit: to provide the system power on/off access with an external dry reed switch. *SW_Sel* signal is used to choose the wireless power switch or the dry reed switch for the capsule
- 2.5 V LDO regulator: to provide power supply to the wireless transceiver, the analog part of the image sensor, and the digital I/O interfaces
- 1.8 V LDO regulator: to provide power supply to the wireless transceiver and the digital part of the image sensor
- 1.2 V LDO regulator: to provide power supply to the digital controller and the wireless transceiver
- 4.0 V charge pump boost regulator: to provide power supply to the strobe flash LEDs
- 24 M crystal oscillator: to provide 24 MHz clock signal to the digital controller (system clock) and the transceiver frequency synthesizer (reference clock)
- 400 MHz wireless transceiver: to transmit image data to the PBS and to receive commands from the PBS
- Digital controller with a customized MCU: to control the system working flow
- CMOS image sensor (CIS) control: to control the image sensor and to acquire image data from the sensor
- JPEG-LS encoder: to perform lossless/near-lossless image compression
- Test mode control: to provide access to SoC internal signals for debug/test purposes

To build the wireless capsule endoscope, the SoC is connected to a CMOS image sensor as shown in Fig. 6.3. The remaining external components include the transceiver antenna, the wireless switch antenna, the dry reed switch, the decoupling capacitors for the regulators, the crystal, and the strobe flash LEDs.

The on-chip LDO regulators can be used to provide power supplies to the function blocks as shown in Fig. 6.4.

WEC SoC Working Flow

The WEC SoC will alternate between the working status and the standby status once switched on. The entire working flow can be divided into six phases, as described below.

Phase I: Initialization

I.0 Power on reset (POR)
I.1 Enable the 20 kHz low frequency/low power RC oscillator to provide clock to the working flow controller and the working flow controller is turned on.
I.2 Enable the on-chip bandgap reference generator, linear LDO regulators one by one.
I.3 Enable the 24 MHz crystal oscillator to provide the system clock to the digital controller.
I.4 The digital controller starts to work.

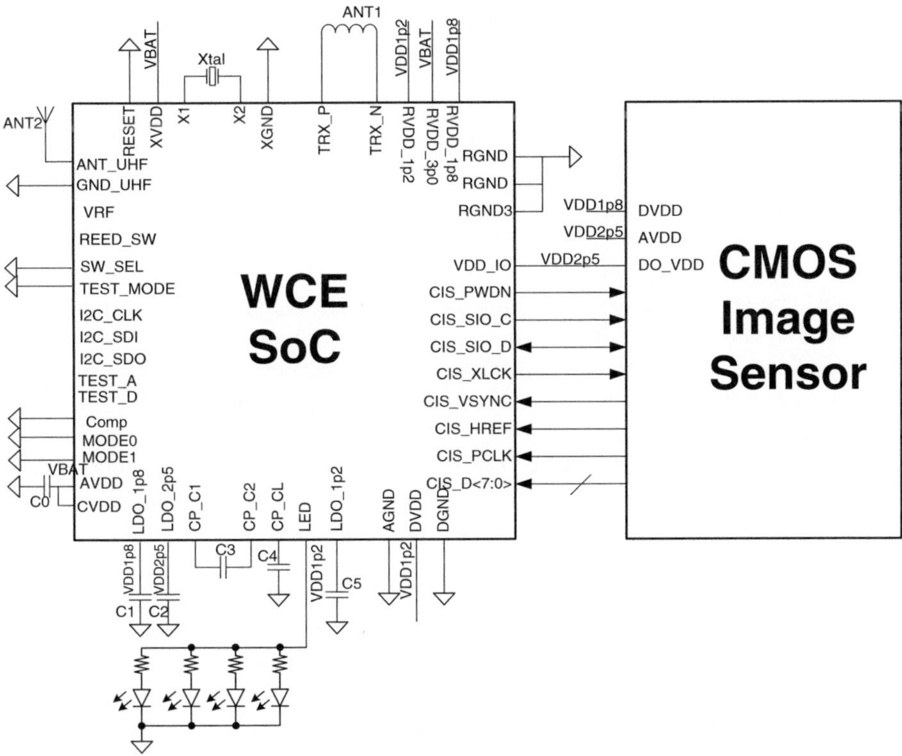

Fig. 6.3 WCE SoC connections in a capsule endoscope

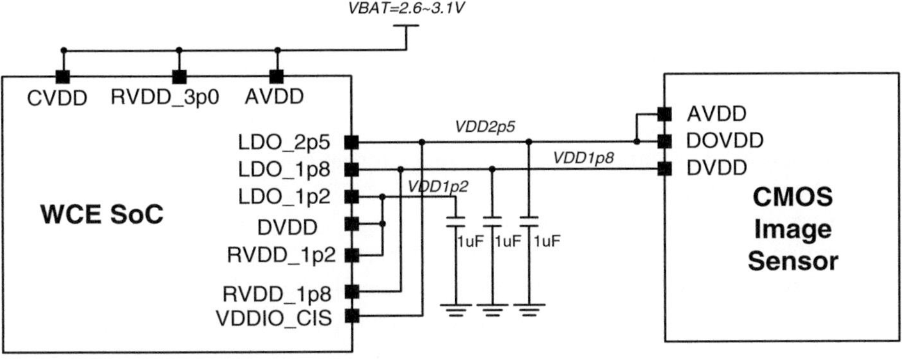

Fig. 6.4 WCE SoC power supply connections

I.5 Enable the calibration circuits for the 20 kHz oscillator and the transceiver, and complete the calibration procedures.

  (a) Calibrate the 20 kHz oscillator.
  (b) Calibrate the VCO in the wireless transceiver synthesizer.
  (c) Calibrate the transceiver antenna port.

I.6 Read from the mode control signal pads.

I.7 Configure the image sensor with default settings.

Phase II: Build Connections with the PBS

II.1 Send notice to the PBS to request configuration commands for 10 ms, and listen to the commands from the PBS for 100 ms. These operations are repeated 30 times. Go to II.4 if commands received from the PBS, or go to II.2 if timeout. The charge pump boost regulator and the strobe flash are turned on when the transmitter is working to give an indication to the user.

II.2 Send notice to the PBS to request configuration commands for 10 ms, listen to the commands from the PBS for 100 ms. If no response from the PBS, wait for 1 s until send notice to the PBS again. These operations are repeated 15 times. Go to II.4 if commands received from the PBS, or go to II.3 if timeout. Again, the charge pump boost regulator and the strobe flash are turned on when the transmitter is working to give an indication to the user.

II.3 Send notice to the PBS to request configuration commands for 10 ms, listen to the commands from the PBS for 100 ms. If no response from the PBS, wait for 5 s until send notice to the PBS again. These operations are repeated until any command is received from the PBS. Go to II.4 if any command is received.

II.4 Validate the command received. Go to II.5 if the command is correct, otherwise return to II.1.

II.5 Go to II.6 if the command contains system configuration information, otherwise go to III.1. (A null command is used as the start signal)

II.6 Perform system configuration according to the command received, and then return to II.1.

Phase III: Image Data Acquisition and Transmission

III.1 Switch on the charge pump boost regulator and the strobe flash LEDs, and then go to III.2.

III.2 Turn on the image sensor, acquire one image, and save it in the on-chip data buffer. If image compression is enabled, perform the image compression during image data acquisition. Go to III.3 when finished.

III.3 Turn off the sensor, the charge pump regulator, and the strobe flash LEDs. Go to III.4 when finished.

III.4 Turn on the transmitter, and wait for 400 μs till the transmitter front-end is settled. The PBS receiver will also have its IF (intermediate frequency) AGC (automatic gain control) settled in this 400 μs. Go to III.5 when finished.

III.5 Pack the image data in the data buffer, and transmit the data packet one by one. Go to III.6 when finished.

III.6 Transmit the continuous waveform (CW) for a certain time period if required, and then go to IV.1

Phase IV: Image Data ARQ (Automatic Repeat-Request)

IV.1 Send notice to the PBS to request ARQ information, and go to IV.2 when finished

IV.2 Listen for the response from the PBS for 100 ms. Go to IV.3 if any command is received, and go to IV.4 if timeout.

IV.3 Validate the command received. Go to IV.5 if correct, otherwise go to IV. 4.

IV.4 Count the number of receiving failures. Go to V.1 if the number exceeds 3, and return to IV.1 if not.

IV.5 Decide whether to perform ARQ according to the command from the PBS. Go to IV. 6 if ARQ is needed, and go to V.1 if ARQ is not needed.

IV.6 Send the wrong image data packets as indicted by the command from the PBS. Return to IV.1 when finished.

Phase V: Reconfigure the Capsule Circuit

This can be done when every N images are transmitted where N can be set by the PBS.

V.1 Determine if it is time to reconfigure the capsule circuit. Go to V.2 if yes, and go to VI if not.

V.2 Send notice to the PBS to request the reconfiguration command. Go to V.3 when finished.

V.3 Listen to the PBS for 100 ms. Go to V.4 if any command is received, and go to V.5 if not.

V.4 Validate the command received from the PBS. Go to V.6 if correct, and go to V.5 if not correct.

V.5 Determine if the number of failures in listening to the PBS exceeds 3. Return to V.2 if not, and go to VI.1 if yes.

V.6 Determine if the PBS requests to reconfigure the capsule circuit. Go to V.7 if yes, and go to VI.1 if not.

V.7 Reconfigure the capsule circuit, and return to V.2 when finished.

Phase VI: Standby

VI.1 Turn off the wireless transceiver.

VI.2 Determine if the time consumed to transmit the current image exceeds the allowed time. Go to VI.3 if not, and go to III.1 if yes.

VI.3 Enter the standby status. The 24 MHz oscillator is turned off during the standby status and only the working flow controller is working using the 20 kHz low frequency clock. Go to III.3 when timeout.

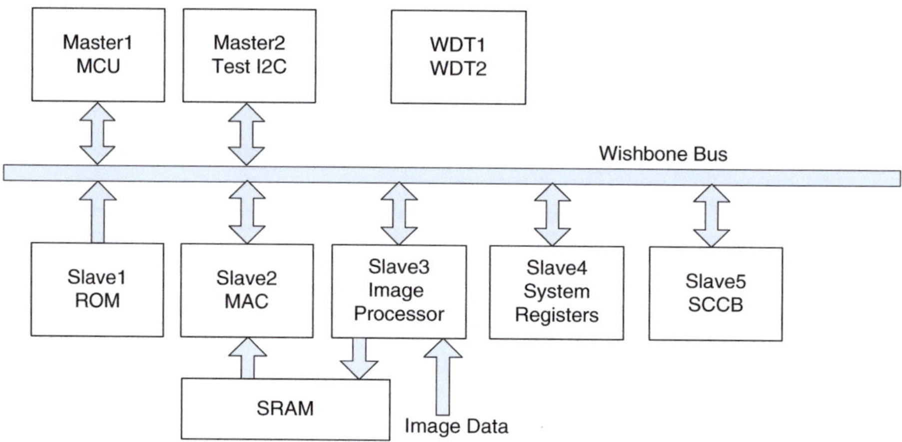

Fig. 6.5 Architecture of the digital controller

Digital Controller

The whole SoC has a ULP digital controller using the architecture presented in Chap. 5, which takes care of system control, image data processing, and the communication protocol. The power management unit and the RF transceiver are controlled by the digital controller as well. The digital controller includes three master modules (including the customized MCU, I^2C controller for test, and the watchdog timer) and six slave modules including the MAC (media access controller), image processor, etc., are connected to the bus as shown in Fig. 6.5.

The customized MCU is the most significant part of the digital controller. It is actually a dedicated low-power control unit with very limited instructions. The high-level MAC protocol is implemented in the program of the MCU, while the real-time image compression and the low-level MAC protocol Fig. 6.6 are accelerated by the specific hardware. This architecture provides adequate function flexibility with high energy efficiency. The techniques of clock-gating and adjustable digital supply voltage are applied to reduce energy dissipation further.

The image processor is a dedicated block which can provide near-lossless image data compression which helps to reduce the data amount to transmit, and consequently to improve the system power efficiency. In this design, the data compression is optional and can be bypassed when needed Fig. 6.6.

Considering the channel noise, the PBS receiver in the application system with a receiving sensitivity of −90 dBm can achieve a raw receiving BER of around 10^{-3}, which is definitely not acceptable for image data transmission. Channel coding is required for the system. In the transmission path, the transmitted data is protected by the cyclic redundancy check (CRC) code and the Reed-Solomon (RS) code, and whitened before transmission. The receiving path has 4B5B decoding, de-whitening, RS decoding, and CRC decoding, correspondingly.

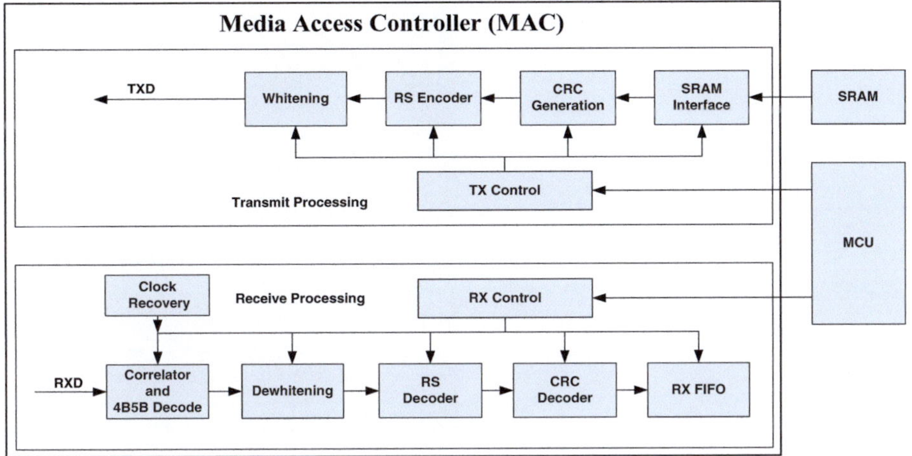

Fig. 6.6 Media access controller

The RS code is chosen to improve the BER from 10^{-3} to 10^{-7}. A BER of 10^{-7} is acceptable when transmitting uncompressed images with 1/4 Mega pixels (480×480). When transmitting compressed images for a higher frame rate, ARQ is utilized to improve the BER further based on the bidirectional communication. Note that the receiver in this SoC consumes higher power than the transmitter, the ARQ scheme is designed such that the receiver is powered on only for the minimal time. For this consideration, data retransmission in used only on a frame base, and the capsule SoC will accept retransmission request from the external data logger only at the end of transmitting each image frame. The implemented ARQ can support a capsule endoscope with 2 fps frame rate even for 480×480 images.

ULP digital circuit design techniques have been adopted to reduce the power consumption of the SoC digital circuit including the image compressor. Clock gating is extensively used as an intrinsic way to implement logic functions and to save power. The flip-flop toggling statistics is gathered at the RTL level of the design and provide early feedback on the effectiveness of clock gating in each function units. Power consumption is re-estimated with actual parasitic extraction using commercial tools at physical implementation level. The simulation results have shown the good correlation of power estimation between RTL and transistor levels. Voltage scaling is another efficient mean to reduce the dynamic power since the power dissipation is proportional to VDD^2. In this SoC power management block, an integrated LDO is applied to provide the supply voltage for the digital controller. The LDO output voltage can be scaled by tuning the LDO feedback network, which is done by the MCU. In the full work mode, the supply voltage is scaled to the predefined value in different phases. The test result shows that the supply voltage can be safely reduced to 1.1 V at image compression phase when 24 MHz clock frequency is applied. To reduce the static power, the supply voltage can be lowered even further and the oscillator can be shut down when the system is disabled.

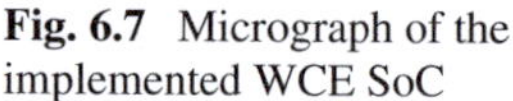

Fig. 6.7 Micrograph of the implemented WCE SoC

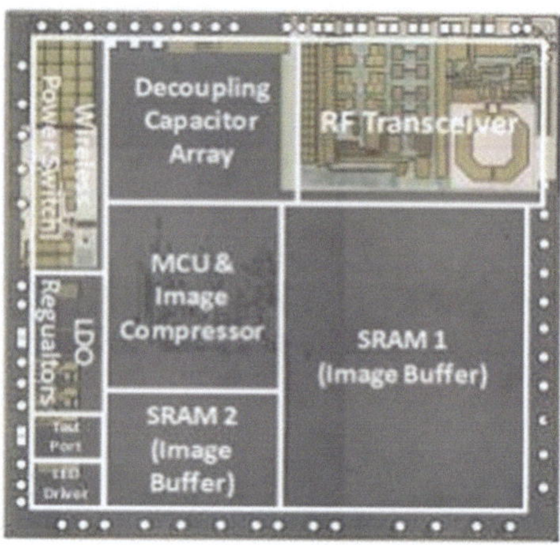

Table 6.1 Capsule endoscope SoC performance summary

Supply voltage		2.5–3.3 V
External components #		7
TX	Type of RF link	Bi-directional
	Bit rate	3 Mbps
	Power consumption	3.9 mW
RX	Bit rate	64 kbps
	Power consumption	12 mW
MCU power consumption		240 µW
Image compressor power		1.1 mW
Image resolution		480×480/240×240
Frame rate		Up to 2 fps @ 480×480 w/compression
Technology		0.18 µm CMOS
Die area		13.3 mm^2

Implementation Results

The SoC has been implemented in 0.18 µm CMOS technology.

The digital controller has 30 k equivalent gates and 94 kB SRAM for image buffering. The die photo of the SoC is shown in Fig. 6.7. It occupies a die area of 13.3 mm^2 (3.7 mm×3.6 mm).

The SoC can work at a voltage down to 2.5 V. The power consumption of the SoC has been checked. The MCU consumes about 200 µA current from a 1.2 V power supply (from the on-chip regulator) when clocked at 24 MHz. The image compressor consumes about 900 µA current from the 1.2 V supply. The MSK transmitter (including all the functional blocks for TX) consumes a total power for 3.9 mW from the 2.5, 1.8, and 1.2 V supplies, while the OOK receiver consumes 12 mW.

The performance of this SoC is summarized in Table 6.1.

Fig. 6.8 Flow to make a
wireless endoscope capsule

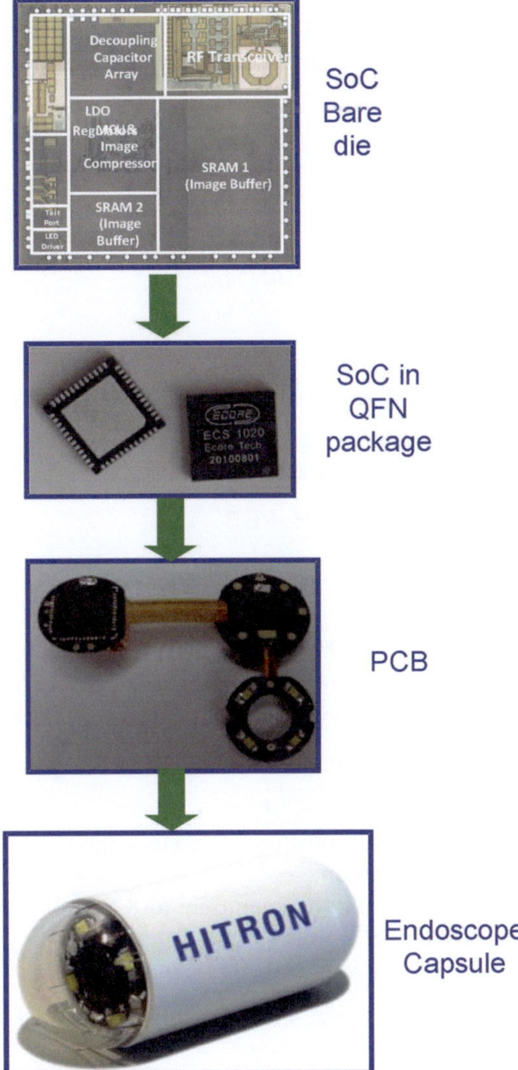

6.1.2   Wireless Capsule Endoscope System

Using the designed WEC SoC, a wireless endoscope capsule is implemented.
Figure 6.8 shows the flow to make an endoscope capsule. Starting from the bare die,
the SoC is first encapsulated in a QFN package. The SoC is assembled on the PCB
on which there are a CMOS image sensor, four strobe flash LEDs, a coil as the
antenna, a crystal, etc. The PCB is then sealed in the capsule shell with the battery
and the optical lens.

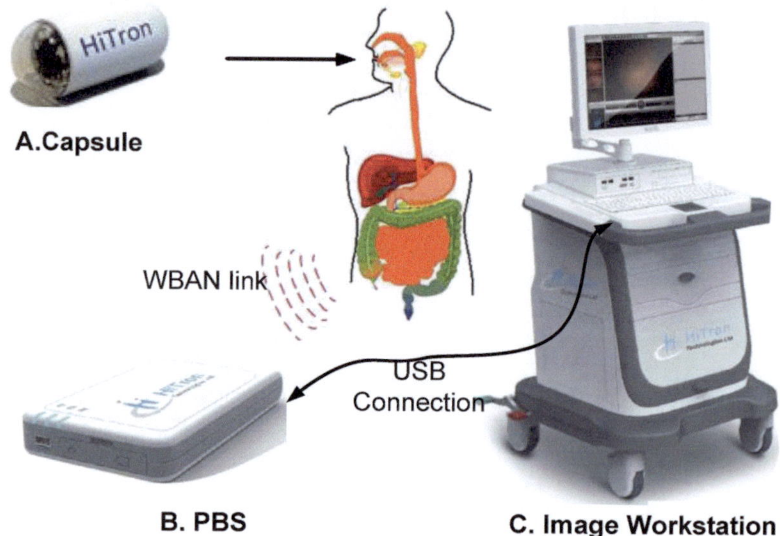

Fig. 6.9 Wireless capsule endoscope system

The entire WCE system includes the capsule, the PBS, and the image workstation. The full set is shown in Fig. 6.9. The product has been cleared by China FDA.
The achieved system performance is summarized as follows:

1. Image resolution: 240×240–480×480, programmable
2. Image frame rate:

   - Image compressor off: up to 4 fps for 240×240 images, and up to 1 fps for 480×480 images
   - Image compressor on: up to 8 fps for 240×240 images and up to 2 fps for 480×480 images

3. Wireless communication: bidirectional
4. Frequency bands: 404–432 MHz, eight channels with 4 MHz intervals
5. Data transmission rate:

   - Raw data rate 1/2/3 Mbps, programmable
   - Effective data rate up to 2 Mbps by subtracting the payload

6. Command receiving data rate: 64 kbps
7. Capsule average current: ≤ 3 mA (TX ≤ 2.5 mA, RX ≤ 7 mA)
8. Capsule leakage current: ≤ 1 μA with dry reed switch, ≤ 0.1 μA with the wireless switch
9. Battery life: ≥ 14 h with 2 1.55 V silver-oxide batteries (82 mAh)

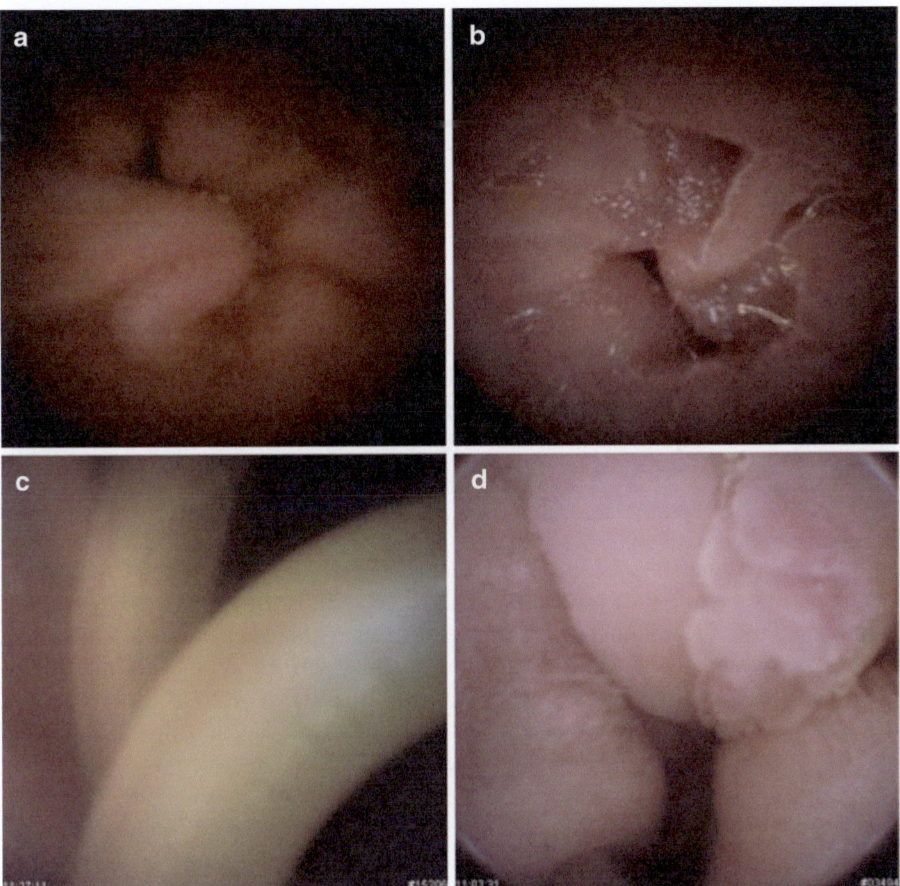

Fig. 6.10 Typical gastrointestinal images taken by the capsule endoscope, (**a**, **b**) good conditions, (**c**) roundworms observed, (**d**) polyps observed

Two human gastrointestinal images are given in Fig. 6.10.

In summary, a ULP SoC has designed for the application of wireless capsule endoscope. The SoC has an RF transceiver working at the 400 MHz UHF band, with a 3 Mbps MSK transmitter and a 64 kbps OOK receiver, enabling the feature of bidirectional communication between the capsule and the external data logger. The MSK transmitter consumes only 3.9 mW power in total. A 1.2 V MCU with a dedicated image compressor and an MAC is implemented to improve the system efficiency. With the SoC, a capsule endoscope can transmit 480×480 images at a frame rate of up to 2 fps. A WCE product using this SoC has been commercialized.

6.2   SoC for Wireless Ligament Balance Measuring in TKA and the Application System

6.2.1   SoC for Wireless Ligament Balance Measuring in TKA

System Overview

Figure 6.11 shows the system architecture of the designed ligament balance measuring system (LBMS) SID. The SID consists of six sensors, an EEPROM and an SoC chip. The sensors are divided into a couple of parts equally. The range of each sensor is 0–1.5 kg, and then the range of each side is 4.5 kg.

For ligament balance measuring, the designed SoC chip acquires the data from the sensors. The acquired sensor data will be processed by the MAC integrated in the SoC chip. The data will be transmitted using the wireless RF transmitter integrated in the SoC chip to the PBS.

The top-level system architecture of the SoC is illustrated in Fig. 6.12. It includes an 8051 microcontroller. EEPROM memories are not available in the CMOS process used to fabricate the chip, and an EEPROM chip is used to store the program bit stream. Once the system powers up, the software is loaded from the EEPROM to the 4 kB on-chip SRAM. The SoC features a serial peripheral interface (SPI). The SPI interface is used to communicate with the EEPROM. A boot-loader block is designed to download the software from the EEPROM. Because the signals collected from the sensors are analog signal, an ADC is needed to convert the analog signal to digital signal. The same wireless transceiver as what used in the WCE SoC is used for this LBMS SoC.

LBMS SoC Implementation

MCU and On-Chip Memory

The core of the SoC digital controller is an MCU based on DW8051 IP core which has higher performance than traditional 8051 microcontroller [7]. The DW8051 IP core

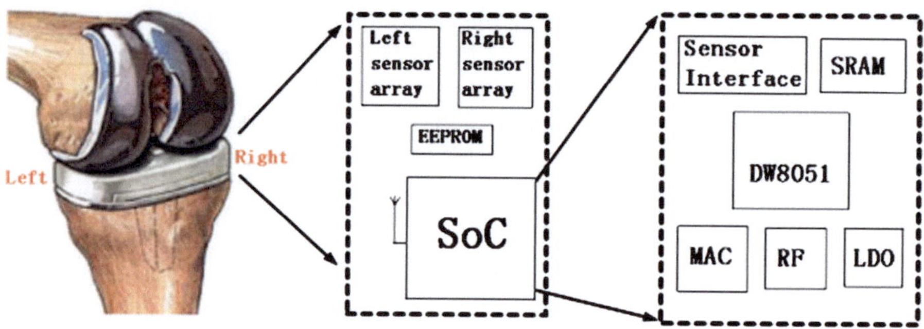

Fig. 6.11   System architecture of LBMS SID

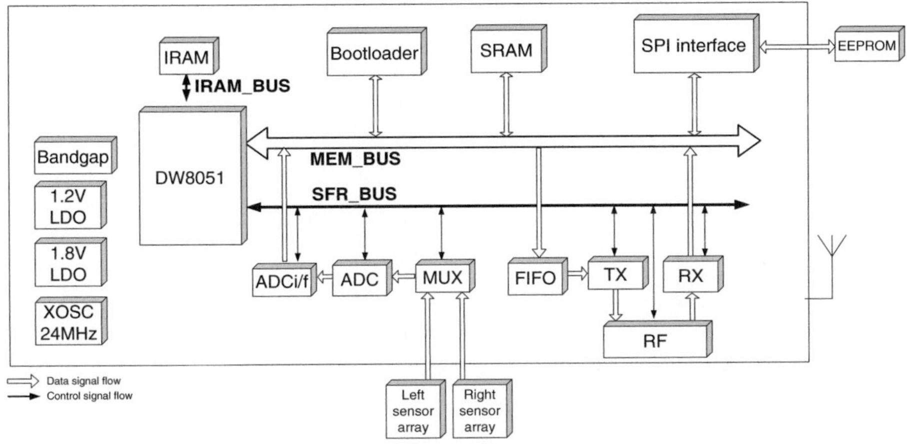

Fig. 6.12 Top-level system architecture of the LBMS SoC

executes each instruction in a 4-clock bus cycle, as opposed to the 12-clock bus cycle in the traditional 8051. And this MCU manages the MAC, SPI interface, ADC interface, and other digital blocks by reading/writing Special Function Registers (SFRs).

The MCU system clock is 12 MHz. The ADC works at 150 kbps and the EEPROM works at 500 kHz. In order to provide the clocks to the ADC and the EEPROM, the clock distribution is designed.

This SoC integrates a 4 kB SRAM and a 256 B SRAM. The size of the SRAM is determined by the recognition task, while the size of the SRAM is determined by the size of program. Because the size of MCU program is less than 4 kB, a 4 kB SRAM would be enough to store the MCU program bit stream. Once the system is powered up, the MCU is initialized. The boot-loader is executed to download the program from the EEPROM to the 4 kB SRAM in the SoC.

MAC and FIFO

The MAC consists of transmission and receiving processing blocks, which is almost identical to that shown in Chap. 5.

FIFO memory is a key component of the SoC, which is commonly used for data buffering and the flow control. A classical asynchronous FIFO is implemented [8]. Asynchronous FIFOs are used to safely pass data from one clock domain to another clock domain. The FIFO designed uses 6-bit pointers with 32 writeable locations to handle full condition, and uses 4-bit pointers with 8 readable locations to help handle empty condition. The data to be written is one byte (8 bits), while the data to be read is four bytes (32 bits). Figure 6.13 shows the full and empty conditions of the FIFO. On reset, both pointers are reset to zero. As soon as the first data is written, the empty flag is cleared. When the write pointer has wrapped around one more time than the read pointer, the FIFO is full. If the high 3 bits of the write pointer is equal to the read pointer, the FIFO is empty.

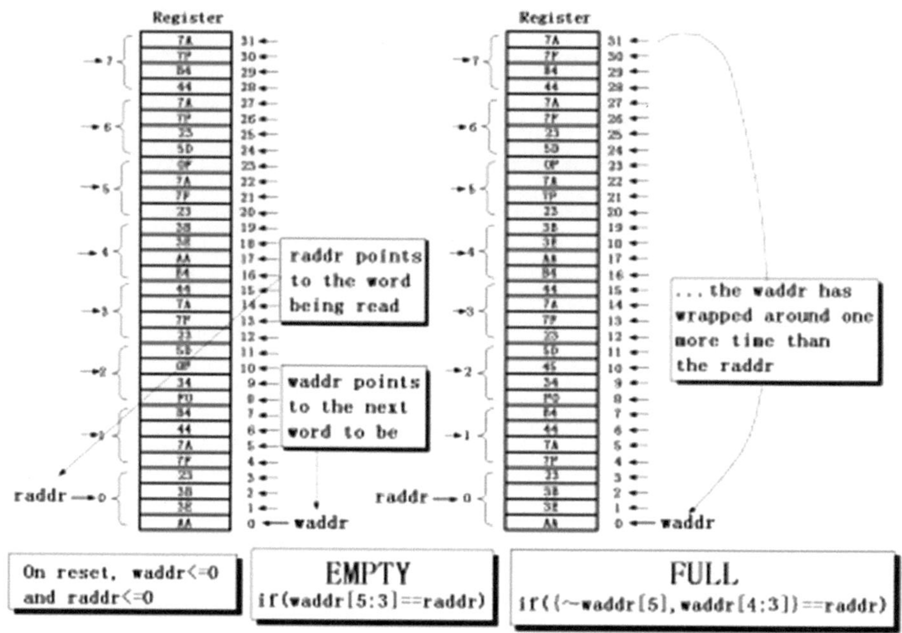

Fig. 6.13 Full and empty conditions of the FIFO

The SoC acquires the data from the sensors one by one. Each data acquired from a single sensor is two bytes. In order to distinguish a sensor from each other, each sensor is marked with a unique label. All the sensors are marked from 0 to 5. As a result, the acquired data will be marked with an additional byte, and the data will be three bytes. For example, the data from the second sensor is $0 \times 1,231$, and the data sent to FIFO will be $0 \times 101,231$. The depth of the FIFO is 32 bytes. If the FIFO is full, an interrupt will be created. At that time, the data of the FIFO will be packaged by the MAC and transmitted by the RF. As soon as the FIFO is not full, the data will continue to be passed to FIFO. Figure 6.14 shows the data processing in this LBMS SoC.

Power Management, RF Transceiver, and ADC

The SoC has three power domains, 3.3 V for the I/O pads, 1.8 V for the digital controller, and 1.2 V for the wireless RF transmitter. Actually, the wireless RF transmitter uses both the 1.2 V and the 1.8 V. There are two LDOs with one converting 3.3–1.8 V and the other converting 3.3–1.2 V. Figure 6.15 shows the power management circuit in this SoC.

The wireless transceiver transmits data using 3 Mbps MSK modulation and receives data using 64 kbps OOK in the half-duplex mode.

The ADC consists of a 4-bit ramp-down converter and a residue amplifier with gain of 2^4. And the power supply voltage is 1.2–3.6 V.

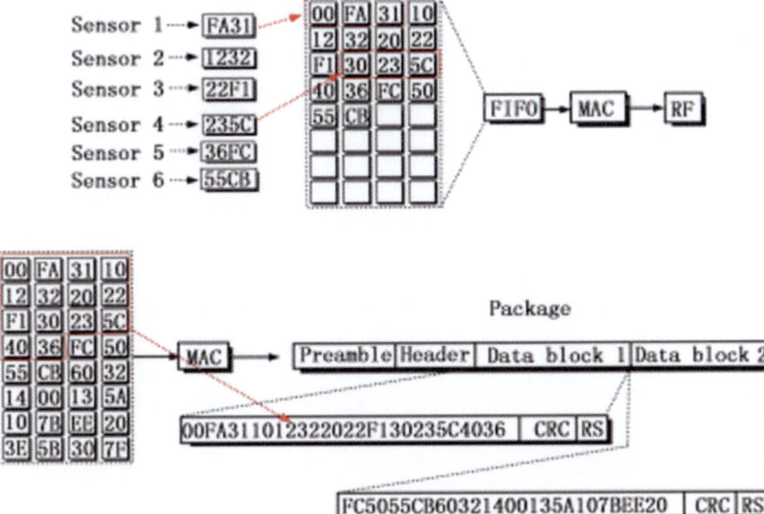

Fig. 6.14 Sensor data processing in LBMS SoC

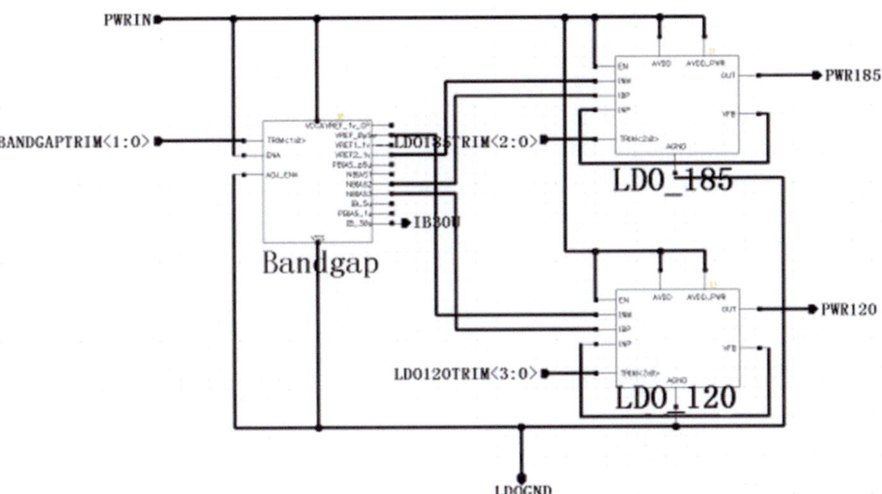

Fig. 6.15 Power management circuit in LBMS SoC

SoC Implementation

The SoC was fabricated in UMC 0.18 μm CMOS technology with a die size of 3 mm×3 mm. The micrograph of the SoC is shown in Fig. 6.16.

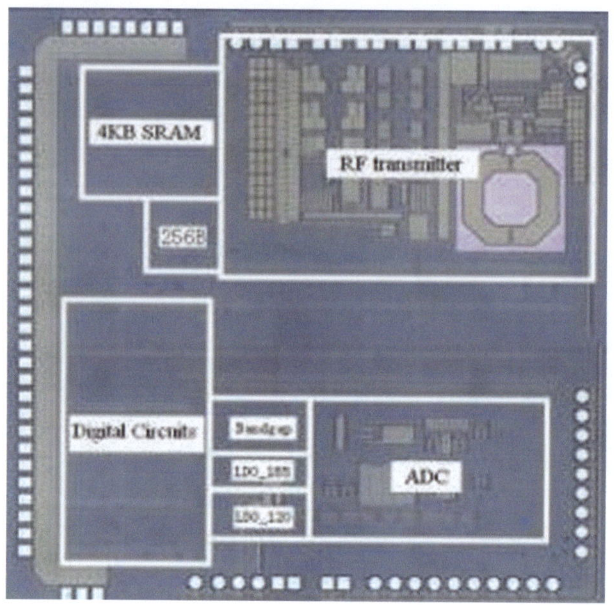

Fig. 6.16 Micrograph of LBMS SoC chip

The test environment for the LBMS SoC is shown in Fig. 6.17, including three boards: the test board with SoC chip (chip on board), the FPGA board with program downloader, and the controller board.

The LBMS SoC performance is summarized in Table 6.2.

6.2.2 Wireless Ligament Balance Measuring System in TKA

Package Design of the LBMS SID

The wireless ligament balance measurement system (LBMS)SID will be used between the femoral component and the tibia component of the artificial implants; the shape of LBMS is designed to match the real spacer of the implants as shown in Fig. 6.18. The package includes upside which embeds eight sensor contact points and underside which holds the printed circuit board (PCB). The sensors touch points are designed to touch the force sensors well with rubber behind to provide the elasticity.

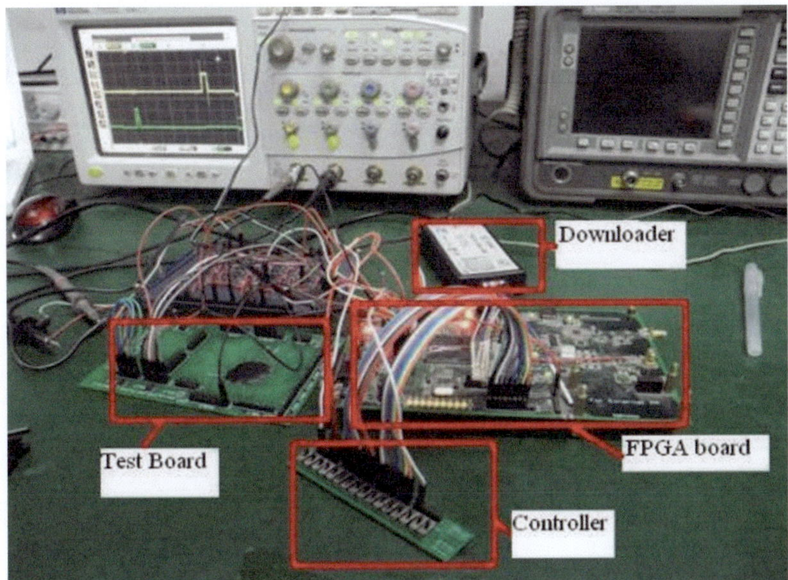

Fig. 6.17   Test environment for the LBMS SoC

Table 6.2   LBMS SoC performance summary

Item	Description
Microcontroller	DW8051
Gate count of digital controller	47,700 gates
Memory	4 kB SRAM, 256 B SRAM
Peripherals	MAC, RF, ADC, MUX, Boot-loader, ADC I/F, FIFO
Fabrication	0.18 μm CMOS process, die size: 3 mm × 3 mm
Supply voltage	1.9–3.6 V
RF channel	404–432 MHz
ADC	16-bit resolution

6.2.3   Lab Experimental Results and Clinic Experiments

Lab experiments were carried out to find whether the system can meet the application requirements. A real human joint from body is used in the experiment as shown in Fig. 6.19. The test results show that the normal unilateral pressure is between 3–5 kg that is under the system linear measurement range (7.5 kg). The two sides of the LBMS have good agreements with the force imposed force. The force corresponding to its distribution is displayed in 3-D in real time with an accuracy of 0.049 N. The proposed system can work properly and display the force data in real time.

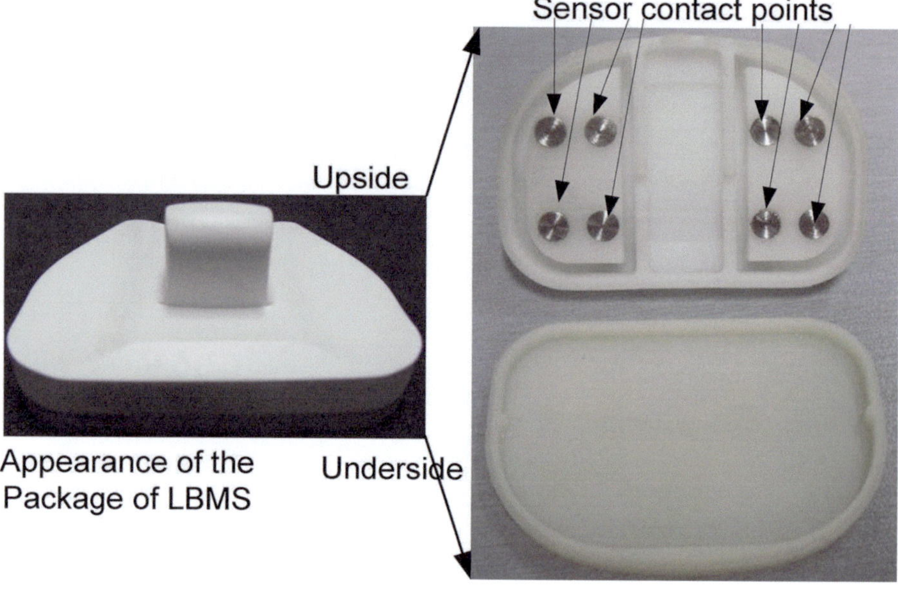

Fig. 6.18 LBMS package SID structure

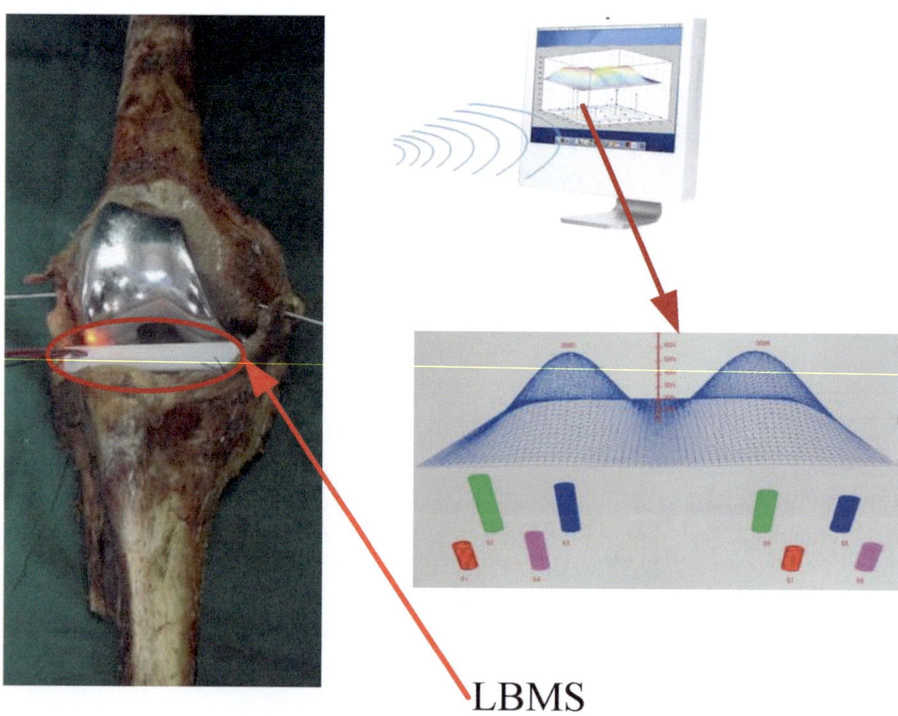

Fig. 6.19 LBMS experimental environment

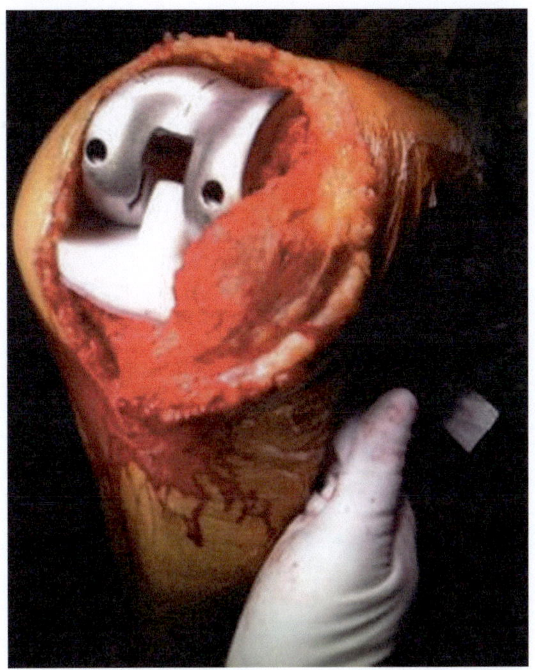

Fig. 6.20 LBMS SID in a clinical experiment

So far about 40 clinical experiments (shown in Fig. 6.20) of the designed LMBS have been carried out in Jishuitan Hospital in Beijing, China. The doctors' feedback shows that the designed system works well and can help surgeons make an accurate judgment on the positions of the artificial knee joint implants.

References

1. Iddan G, Meron G, Glukhovsky A, et al. Wireless capsule endoscopy. Nature. 2000;405:417–8.
2. Given Imaging, overview of products. http://www.givenimaging.com/en-us/Patients/Pages/pageSmallBowel.aspx
3. Olympus. Olympus launches high-resolution capsule endoscope in Europe. http://www.olympus-global.com/en/news/2005b/nr051013capsle.html
4. P. Bradley. RF integrated circuits for medical implants: meeting the challenge of ultra low-power. http://www.cmoset.com/uploads/Peter_Bradley.pdf
5. Chen X, Zhang X, Zhang L, Li X, Qi N, Jiang H, Wang Z. A wireless capsule endoscope system with low-power controlling and processing asic. IEEE Trans Biomed Circuits Syst. 2009;3(1):11–22.
6. Xie X, Li G, Chen X, Li X, Wang Z. A low-power digital IC design inside the wireless endoscopic capsule. IEEE Journal of Solid-State Circuits. 2006;41(11):2390–400.

7. Liu M, Chen H, Zhang C, ChangMeng L, Wang Z. A light-powered sub-threshold microprocessor. J Semicond. 2010;31(11):1150021–6.
8. Xu Zhang, Hong Chen, Ming Liu, Hanjun Jiang, Chun Zhang and Zhihua Wang. Sensor interface with single-line quasi-digital output for ligament balance measuring system. International Conference on Biomedical circuits and systems (BIOCAS2011), San Diego, CA; 2011. p. 377–380

Summary

A typical wireless medical/health care system is composed of the remote side and the local side. The remote side, which provides medical/health information service, includes the data service center, the hospitals, and the doctors. The local side is the equipment carried by the users, which is composed of the PBS (portable base station) and the SIDs (sensing/intervention devices). The CMOS integrated circuit design techniques discussed in this book are mainly for the SIDs.

In addition to the regular performance parameters, such as the accuracy, speed, signal-to-noise ratio, linearity, and stability, the SIDs have some special requirements, to work in/around the human bodies. The two most important performances for SIDs are the form factor and the battery life. To meet these two requirements, the IC designed for the SIDs have two special design specs, the integration level and the power consumption. The circuit design techniques presented in this book mainly focus on how to minimize the power consumption both at the circuit block level and the system level, and how to improve the IC integration level such that the external components' count is as small as possible.

1. The biomedical sensor acquisition circuits: the biomedical sensor output signal usually has very limited bandwidth; the interface circuit and the digitization circuit should be designed to match the signal characteristics. Particularly, to save power consumption, the circuit should not be over-designed in terms of speed and accuracy. To further save power, the designers should try some unconventional circuit structures other than the commonly used circuit types, such as the voltage-to-pulse converter in contrast to the traditional ADC as introduced in Chap. 3.
2. The wireless transceivers: the wireless transceiver usually consumes most part of the total energy in an SID. To save the power consumption by transceivers, the system should first be optimized. For example, in the capsule endoscope, an image data compressor is included to reduce the total data amount such that the data transmission power can be greatly saved. A good trade-off between the power consumption and other performances should be made for the SID transceiver. It should be noted that many existing transceivers available on market

Z. Wang et al., *CMOS IC Design for Wireless Medical and Health Care,*
DOI 10.1007/978-1-4614-9503-1, © Springer Science+Business Media New York 2014

have excessive performances for SIDs, such as the output signal level and networking complexity. The best solution for SIDs is to design application-optimized transceiver, such as the circuits presented in Chap. 4.

3. The power management circuits: for SIDs with extreme requirement on the form factor, it is necessary to implement the power management unit on-chip. As shown in Chap. 5, a power supply scheme should be carefully designed, such as what we have done in the capsule endoscope SoC. To further overcome the bottleneck, other power techniques, such as the wireless energy transfer and the energy harvesting, should be taken into consideration.

4. The digital controller: to design a low power digital controller for SIDs, a good solution is to use a customized MCU plus some hard accelerators for some specific functions, as shown in Chap. 5. The MCU can be optimized by simplifying the instruction set. Such architecture can help to accomplish the SID flow control and signal processing functions with adequate implementation flexibility under affordable power consumption.

5. SoC: the system-on-a-chip is the best solution for SIDs with very stringent form factor requirement. The design examples of the two SoCs for the specific applications using the circuit techniques presented in previous chapters have been given in Chap. 6, which can provide some hints for the readers when implementing similar systems.

In summary, the CMOS circuit design techniques for the wireless capsule endoscope and the wireless ligament measurement system in TKA have been presented. The system level design considerations, the SoC architectures and the SoC level optimization, the transistor-level details of the function blocks, as well as the implementation results have been discussed in this book. The contents included in this book can be used as reference for designing the low power wireless medical and health care application systems.

We believe that with the continuous effort from the industry and academia on the area of wireless medical and health care techniques, the people will finally reach a status in which the medical and health care becomes available for everybody at anytime, anywhere. We will finally see that the current sickness-oriented medical/health care becomes prevention-oriented service, and the quality of life can be further greatly improved.

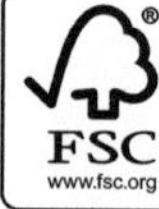
MIX
Papier aus verantwortungsvollen Quellen
Paper from responsible sources
FSC® C105338

If you have any concerns about our products,
you can contact us on
ProductSafety@springernature.com

In case Publisher is established outside the EU,
the EU authorized representative is:
Springer Nature Customer Service Center GmbH
Europaplatz 3, 69115 Heidelberg, Germany

Printed by Libri Plureos GmbH
in Hamburg, Germany